ABS OF STEEL ™

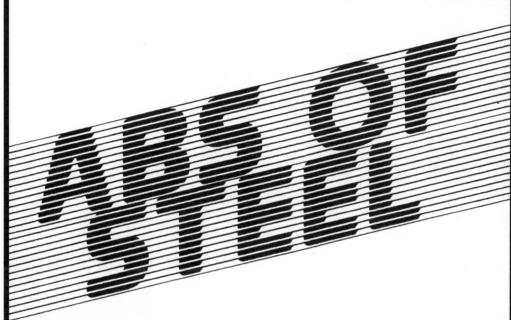

Flatter, Firmer Abs in Just Four Weeks

LEISA HART & LIZ NEPORENT, M.A.

SUMMIT PUBLISHING GROUP

THE SUMMIT PUBLISHING GROUP
One Arlington Centre, 1112 East Copeland Road, Fifth Floor
Arlington, Texas 76011

Printed in the United States of America

99 98 97 96 95   1 2 3 4 5

Hart, Leisa.
    Abs of steel : flatter, firmer abs in just four weeks / by Leisa Hart and
Liz Neporent.
        p. cm.
    Includes index.
    ISBN 1-56530-183-8 (alk. paper)
    1. Exercise for women. 2. Abdomen—Muscles. I. Neporent, Liz.
II. Title.
GV508.H37 1996
613.7′1—dc20   95-47797
                                                     CIP

Cover Photo by Don Banks
Photography by Truitt Rogers
Illustrations by Peter Fan

Acknowledgments

To Liz Neporent, Melissa Berman, Eve Silverman, Cecilia Parks, Jordan Woy, Len Oszustowicz, and especially my parents

LEISA HART

To my husband, Jay Shafran, Leisa Hart, Holly Byrne, Bob Welter, Terry Certain, Debbie Benazzi, Patti Buttenheim, Deb Dennis, Lisa Swain, Mia Holt-Heller, and especially my family

LIZ NEPORENT

Table of Contents

Foreword

After more than twenty-five years as an exercise researcher and fitness specialist, the most frequent question I hear is, "How can I get rid of this?" while the asker points to his or her midsection area. In our affluent society we experience an undesirable effect from too much food and too little physical activity, namely the accumulation of body fat. Typically, much of the fat is stored in the midsection area, which leads to other problems. One is an unattractive personal appearance, another is excess stress on the vulnerable lower-back area, and a third is a greater risk of cardiovascular disease.

Of course, the solution to this problem is not as simple as a few trunk curls to tighten, tone, and trim the abdominal region. More physical activity, better eating habits, regular aerobic exercise, and some strength training may all be helpful in losing fat and gaining fitness. However, a specific contingent of conditioning exercises for the abdominal and lower back muscles is certainly the key to a firm, functional, and attractive midsection.

Liz Neporent's and Leisa Hart's approach to abdominal training in *Abs of Steel* provides a well-designed and strategically developed program of strengthening and stretching exercises for all of the midsection muscles. The chapters that address the *rectus abdominis* muscles, *internal/external oblique* muscles, and *erector spinae* muscles are superb. They present the anatomy and function of these important muscles and provide safe and productive exercises for conditioning them in a comprehensive and progressive manner.

The actual training process is the key to midsection fitness, and this is where Liz Neporent's and Leisa Hart's exercise expertise really makes the difference. The *Abs of Steel* training protocol is based on sound principles of muscle strengthening and stretching, principles that ensure effective and efficient exercise, rather than countless repetitions of unproductive movements. The emphasis is to make every exercise and every repetition count, and this is the right approach to maximize results with relatively brief training sessions.

Abs of Steel provides progressive training programs that address all levels of midsection conditioning. The self-tests make it easy to identify your present abilities, and the variety of exercises enhances both motivation and results. Perhaps most important, the comprehensive approach to strengthening and stretching all of the midsection muscles ensures increased physical fitness and decreased injury risk as well as a better personal appearance.

In the final analysis, *Abs of Steel* is a remarkably insightful book that provides a highly practical and successful approach to midsection conditioning. In addition to the technical soundness of this text, it is easy to read and understand. The information is precise, the writing style is concise, and the person who practices the *Abs of Steel* program should soon see some serious midsection improvement.

Wayne L. Westcott, Ph.D., is a fitness researcher and author of four college textbooks on strength training.

Introduction

Abs Of Steel: The Revolutionary Approach to Abdominal Training

You probably selected this book because you are interested in improving your appearance, and you know that firm, defined abdominals are the centerpiece of any fit body. You may also know from doing our exercise videos that *Abs of Steel* is one of the most results-oriented abdominal training programs around.

This book will teach you safe, adaptable, exercises, routines, and techniques especially designed to tighten your middle. You'll learn countless ways to customize your program to suit your needs and preferences as well as improve your fitness level. The information you will find on these pages will give you the ability to revise your routine every time you need a change. You'll learn the best way to improve quickly—and keep on improving!

As you read through the chapters that follow, you will notice something unique for a book about abdominals. We do not refer to our program as simply abdominal training, rather, we refer to it as *Abs of Steel* middle-muscle training. That's because this program thoroughly works *all* of the muscles which wrap around your middle and give it shape. You will learn to work all of your middle muscles together as a team, just as they function in everyday life, plus you'll learn to target tone each individual muscle group with special isolation exercises.

Think of middle-muscle training as a three-dimensional approach to firming up your middle. "Traditional" abdominal programs are one-dimensional, usually centered on doing some type of "crunch," "curl-up," or "sit-up" movements. While crunches are an important part of any abdominal strengthening and toning regimen, they only stress a few muscles and address only one type of movement your middle is capable of performing. No wonder you feel dissatisfied with the results of typical abdominal workouts, even if you follow them to the letter. *Abs of Steel* middle-muscle training takes into account the fact that your torso has a front, a back, and sides! You work all of your middle muscles completely and in a variety of ways so you'll look good from every angle. You will see dramatic results more quickly than you've ever dreamed possible. Aesthetics aside, this is the best way to develop good posture and a strong, flexible, pain-free lower back.

Abs of Steel middle-muscle training is also superior to most other abdominal training systems because of our emphasis on technique. When it comes to proper form, you are usually left in the dark by other programs. That's why you often wind up with a sore neck or a throbbing backache and not much improvement in your abdominal muscles to show for your efforts. *Abs of Steel* training provides very clear, specific directions on how to correctly exercise your middle muscles. It's very complete, extremely precise, and ultimately, the most effective way to strengthen and tone your middle.

One other important difference between *Abs of Steel* training and most other abdominal work: it doesn't waste your time. Many traditional abdominal training systems call for you to perform hundreds or even thousands of repetitions per workout. Consequently, working your abs becomes a very time-consuming task. *Abs of Steel* can give you results in as little as five minutes per workout. That's just fifteen minutes a week. How is this possible? Because our middle-muscle training system makes every repetition

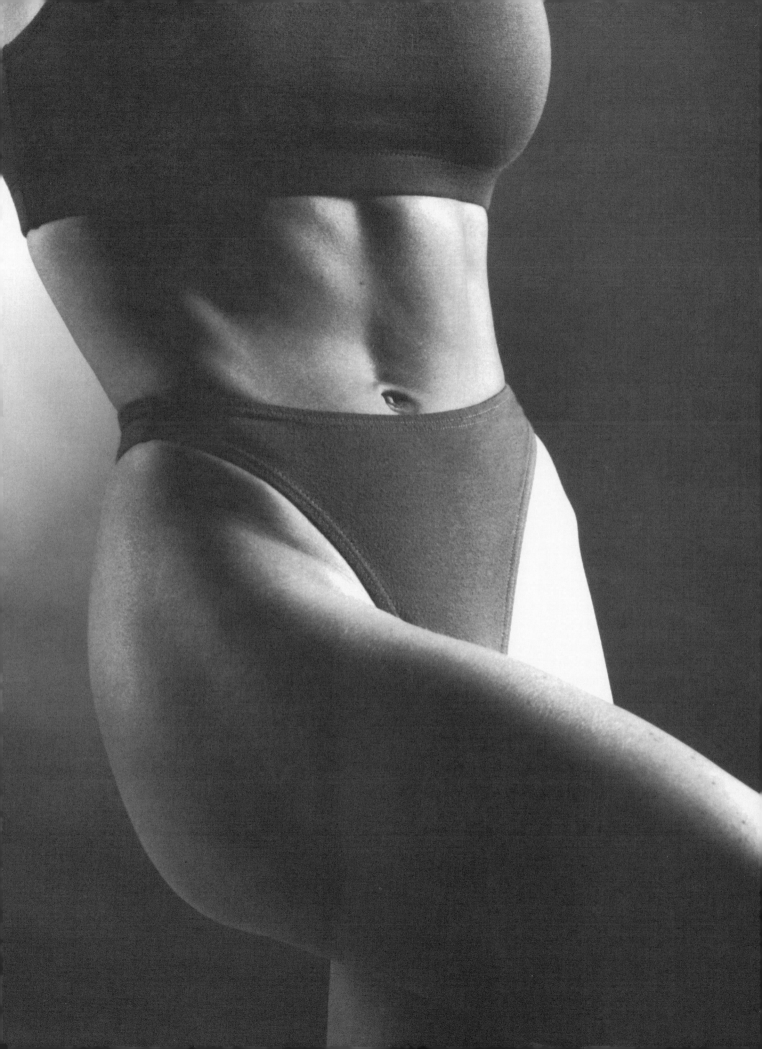

count. Our belief is that if you can do hundreds of reps of an exercise, it isn't intense enough or precise enough to produce positive changes in your middle muscles. We have designed exercises and techniques that are amazingly effective, and then we have arranged them in a specific order to give you even better results. You will see significant improvement by doing as few as five repetitions of some exercises and as few as four exercises per workout.

No matter what, you'll never do more than twenty-five repetitions of any move. Once you can do that many repetitions easily and with proper form, you'll make the exercise more challenging by changing one or more of the *Abs of Steel* training variables described in the following chapters or by doing a more difficult routine. Imagine that. Beautifully sculpted abs and still enough time left over to show them off!

We hope you enjoy your *Abs of Steel* training as much as we enjoy bringing it to you. We know that if you follow our advice you can create a slimmer, firmer, shapelier middle.

Oh, and there's one more thing: in our bonus *Buns of Steel* chapter at the end of this book (p. 94), you'll find eight of the best buns sculpting exercises you have ever tried. You'll also find buns routines for every exercise level and variations to make each move more challenging and interesting. After all, nothing else complements *Abs of Steel* like *Buns of Steel*!

Good luck and have a great workout!

Chapter 1

The Abs of Steel Middle-Muscle Training System

Brief Anatomy Lesson

You are probably used to thinking of your "tummy" as the area to exercise if your goal is a flat, toned midsection. After all, that's what you see every time you face a mirror. But if that's the only part of your midriff you ever work, you will find it difficult to develop true "Abs of Steel."

You didn't know there was more than one muscle group surrounding and shaping your middle? Well then, let's take the time to review both the location and function of the five muscles collectively referred to in the **Abs of Steel** training system as your middle muscles.

To begin with, all of your middle muscles have something in common: they are all responsible for the movement and stabilization of your spine. Your middle body moves in a variety of ways; it can bend, twist, arch, round, or simply hold still while you move your arms and legs. The unique design of your spine and the muscles that attach to it make this remarkable complexity of movement possible.

Your spine consists of twenty-four individual bones called vertebrae, stacked one on top of the other like a series of neatly piled building blocks. It has three distinct curves and runs the length of your torso. Each vertebra is capable of only a small amount of movement but the combined motion of all of them provides you with wide ranging mobility. Your middle muscles act like ropes which pull on levers (your vertebrae) to move your spine.

Your *rectus abdominis* is the muscle you are probably referring to whenever you speak about your "abs" or "stomach." It's the muscle that spans the length and width of your middle body, attaching below your breastbone and onto your pelvis. Incidentally, it's not correct to refer to this muscle, or any other muscle, as your stomach. Your stomach is the organ used for digesting food. Your *rectus* is the muscle that initiates spinal movement. Your *rectus* is responsible for flexing your spine—in other words, any forward bending, curling, or crunching movement.

Your *internal* and *external obliques* are the abdominal muscles closest to the surface. In addition to aiding your *rectus* in the flexing of your spine, they're used for twisting and side-bending movements. Your *external obliques* originate at the side of your lower ribs, run diagonally across your torso, and attach onto the fibrous edges of your *rectus abdominis* muscle. Your *internal obliques* run at right angles to, and underneath, the *external obliques*.

The muscles that attach to the back of your spine are known as the *erector spinae*. They extend, or arch, your spine backward.

Your *transversus abdominis* runs underneath your *rectus*. Though it doesn't control any spinal action, it assists all of your other muscles in stabilizing, or supporting, your spine. Stabilization is a very important function of your middle muscles. Adequate stabilization is important for good posture, flat abs, proper breathing, and injury prevention.

The System

The **Abs of Steel** training system works your middle with exercises that isolate each individual muscle as well as work them

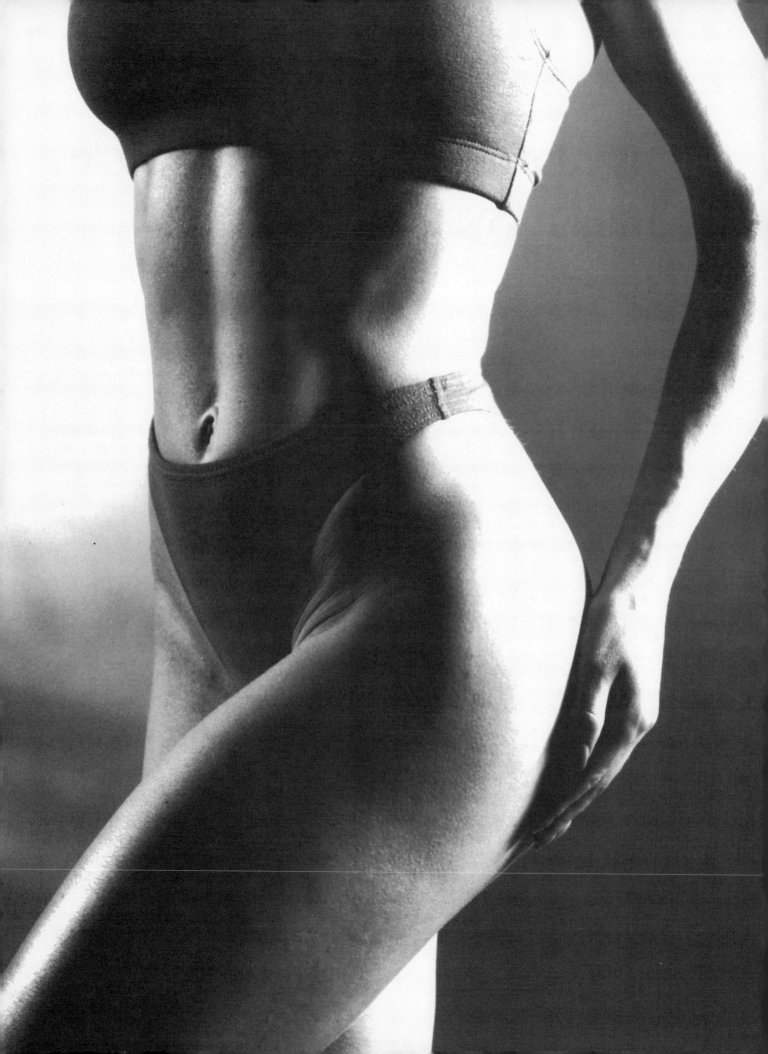

together, as a team. This is the most complete approach to middle-muscle training you can do—and it is why no other method will give you better results than **Abs of Steel.**

You will do five types of exercises in the **Abs of Steel** training system. This may seem like a lot at first, but you actually can get results by doing as few as four strengthening exercises per workout—about five minutes of training. As long as you regularly include at least one exercise of each type (plus a postworkout stretch), you get complete muscle usage and faster, better results.

- *Stabilization and Awareness*: These exercises work all of your middle muscles simultaneously. They teach them how to function together as they must in everyday life and teach you how it feels when you are using your muscles correctly, both during exercise and in typical, real-life situations.

  Stabilization and awareness exercises are done at the beginning of every **Abs of Steel** routine as a reminder of correct usage and form when doing the exercises that follow. They also thoroughly warm up all of your middle muscles.

- *Lower-Back Training*: Because your lower-back muscles are prone to weakness and tightness, it's important to keep them both strong and supple. Accordingly, half of the lower-back exercises in this book stretch your back extensor muscles; the other half strengthen them. Doing your lower-back training right after stabilization and awareness while these muscles are not yet tired helps avoid injury and overuse.

- *Abdominal Training*: Next up in the **Abs of Steel** sequence are exercises designed to isolate your *rectus* and *transversus abdominals*. These include all crunch-type movements, the typical "meat-and-potatoes" of most abdominal training programs. These are the exercises that flatten, tighten, and tone your tummy.

- *Waist Training*: The last group of strengthening exercises zeros in on your *internal and external obliques*. All of these exercises involve rotation, twisting, or bending. They complete the middle-muscle, target-toning series. By exhausting all of your other middle-muscle groups first, you will get true oblique isolation.

- *Stretching Out:* A loose, limber spine contributes to perfect posture and helps you benefit the most from the strengthening exercises. Although your stretching exercises are not listed as part of the **Abs of Steel** routines, they are still vital to your program's success. Strength work should always be balanced with some sort of flexibility work, usually at the end of your workout. Our stretching series provides a complete total body stretch with an emphasis on the muscles that tend to get tight and sore from middle-muscle training.

Training Variables

To get results from target toning, you must constantly challenge the muscle being worked. Muscles quickly adapt to stress placed upon them by growing stronger and firmer.

When you target tone most muscles, you typically add an external resistance such as a free weight, a weight machine, or an exercise band to increase the intensity and effectiveness of the exercise. Unfortunately, this is not a practical method to use to develop your middle muscles. Although you can add resistance to some middle-muscle exercises, only very advanced exercisers can handle this technique, and even then only in limited amounts. (See *Breaking Out of Your Routine*, p. 88.) Most exercisers will find it awkward or downright uncomfortable to do a middle-muscle exercise while holding a weight.

In lieu of added resistance, the **Abs of Steel** middle-muscle training system offers you ways to challenge your muscles with variety. There are virtually unlimited techniques for varying your program. Simply adjust one or more of the following training variables:

- *Exercise:* Though all the moves of the same type have a similar focus, each works your muscles in a slightly different way by either changing the angle or emphasizing a different part of the muscle. Changing the exercises you do on a frequent basis keeps your muscles off balance: since they never have time to get used to any one stimulus, they must constantly adapt, strengthen, tone, and tighten.

- *Exercise Variations*: We offer at least one variation for every exercise in this book. Some make the move harder; some make it easier. Additionally, there are several other special advanced techniques for varying the exercises in *Breaking Out of Your Routine* (p. 88).

- *Repetitions:* A repetition is one complete movement of an exercise. You can increase the number of "reps" you do to make an exercise harder, or decrease the number of reps to make it easier.
- *Sets:* A set is a group of repetitions. Increasing the number of sets of an exercise makes the overall routine more difficult.
- *Rest:* The more rest you take between sets, the less intense the workout. You should take enough time to allow your muscles to regain strength for the next set, but not so much time that you lose your focus. The stronger your muscles become, the less rest you will need between sets. Rest also refers to time between workouts. In general, you should rest at least one day between workouts for a particular muscle group to allow it time to repair and recoup.

Your middle muscles will thrive on change, so do adjust your training variables frequently. It's not wise to change more than two training variables per workout. If you do, it may result in overtraining, burnout, or injury.

Precise, Thorough Movement

Another way the ***Abs of Steel*** training system ensures dramatic results is by emphasizing *quality* of movement over *quantity* of movement. While many other abdominal workout programs will have you doing hundreds of time-consuming reps, our program has you doing between five and twenty repetitions while emphasizing perfect form. You will spend less time training and more time showing off your flat, streamlined middle!

Although every group of exercises in the ***Abs of Steel*** program focuses on a different middle muscle and a different movement of your spine, many of the basic form points apply to all the exercises. Many of these will be covered in both the *Set-Up, Move,* and *Form Tips* section of each exercise description. Pay attention to these sections. Read them carefully and follow them to the letter. They will make all the difference between simply doing an exercise and doing it right.

Meanwhile, let's go over some of the basic form

and technique points in detail. You should review this section from time to time so that perfect form remains a top training priority.

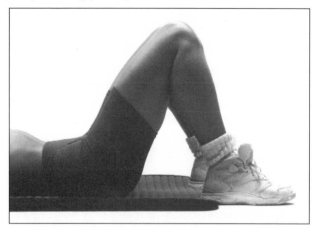

- *Anchoring (see above):* When you lie on your back to do an exercise, pull your abs inward toward your spine and press your back into the floor. This protects your lower back from injury and engages all of your middle muscles. When you stand, sit, kneel, or lie on your stomach, you should also pull your abs inward. (The Slide and Extended Contraction found in the *Stabilization and Awareness* chapter, p. 16, are excellent exercises for practicing and understanding this form point.)

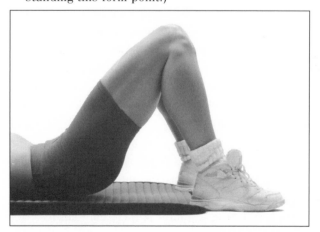

- *Pelvic Tilt (see above)*: The *Pelvic Tilt* is an exercise in and of itself; you'll find it in the *Lower Back* chapter (p. 28). Pelvic tilting during an exercise, brings your spine into proper alignment and further pulls all of your middle muscles in toward your spine. When doing a back exercise while in a prone position, tilt your pelvis slightly upward by gently squeezing your buns together and curling your spine so your buns lift slightly off the floor. Your lower back remains firmly anchored into the floor.

For exercises where you are lying on your stomach, pull your abs inward and tilt your pelvis as if you're trying to create a small space between your navel and the floor.

- *Alignment:* All exercises call for good spinal alignment. Your spine should form a straight line from your neck to your tailbone. In doing these exercises, you should not attempt to eliminate the natural curves of your back and neck.

- *Breathing:* Always exhale forcefully through your mouth during the effort phase of an exercise (exertion) and inhale deeply through your nose as you move into the relaxation phase. (For most exercises this means exhaling as you lift and inhaling as you lower.)

Proper breathing fully engages your middle muscles and speeds oxygen-rich blood into your working muscles. Holding your breath can cause sharp changes in your blood pressure, which could lead to premature fatigue, dizziness, and fainting.

- *Quality of Movement*: We can't overstate the importance of this factor. All **Abs of Steel** movements should be done slowly and with control. Never rush through an exercise by bouncing, jerking, or snapping your body from one position to the next. Take the time to feel each and every repetition. Concentrate on engaging the muscle you're working so you can feel it contract and relax. Rely on muscle, not momentum.

A Word About Total Fitness

Working your middle muscles is an important part of overall fitness, but it's certainly not the whole picture. A body that is in top form is the ideal showcase for your flat, contoured tummy. Optimal fitness is really the sum of four parts: whole body strength, cardiovascular endurance, flexibility, and nutrition. Here's some important information about these four factors:

- *Whole Body Strength*: Strength training not only keeps your muscles strong, it also helps you maintain a healthy weight. Because muscle is very active tissue, it burns up more calories than body fat, so you can eat more without gaining weight. And

because muscle is denser, it takes up less room than fat. When you gain muscle, you lose inches without losing much scale weight. (You can check out the *Buns of Steel Total Body Workout* for more on strength training and target toning.)

It's advisable to maintain a desirable fat-to-muscle ratio, often referred to as *body fat percentage*. For women, an optimal body fat percentage is between 16 and 26 percent; for men, between 12 and 20 percent. A healthy amount of body fat lets your muscle definition show through.

Strength training in general, and target toning in particular, can solve many of your physique flaws. You can't spot reduce—selectively lose fat in a particular area—but you can reshape an area. Strength training makes a muscle firmer, tighter, and more toned. You can improve upon nature by reproportioning your body with regular target-toning sessions.

One set of strength training for each major muscle group done at least twice a week will reward you with the benefits of increased strength, maintained bone density, and a firmer, shapelier appearance. Major muscle groups include your upper back, chest, shoulders, arms, buns, legs, and of course, your middle muscles. Use a moderate weight (or intensity); one that stresses your muscles yet allows you to do 12-20 reps with proper form.

- *Cardiovascular Exercise*: Cardiovascular, or aerobic exercise, refers to any sustained, rhythmic activity done with your larger muscle groups. Activities such as walking, jogging, and cycling fall into this category. Anything that gets your heart rate pumping and makes you breathe hard for a period of twenty minutes or more qualifies.

Cardiovascular exercise will burn calories and help you shed unwanted body fat. What all the aerobic exercise in the world *won't* do is help you shape your body into the form you've always wanted. For that, you need target toning.

Performed on a regular basis, cardiovascular exercise will improve your stamina for fitness, sports, and daily activities. It will lower your blood pressure, cholesterol, and stress levels. And, as research has overwhelmingly shown, it can be an invaluable tool for preventing, and helping individuals recover from, heart disease.

In order to achieve a reasonably good level of fitness, you must do a minimum of three twenty-minute sessions a week. If your goal is weight loss and body fat reduction, you'll need to do more.

To be effective, all aerobic exercise should get your heart rate into its target heart rate zone (THZ). You can determine your THZ by subtracting your age from 226 and then multiplying the result by .6 to find the low end of your range and .8 to find the high end of your range. When you exercise, your heart should be beating within this range.

Check your heart rate, or pulse, approximately every fifteen minutes or during the peak intensity of your workout. You can do this by placing two fingers on your wrist directly below your thumb, counting the number of beats you feel in six seconds, and then multiplying this number by four. (Better yet, wear a heart rate monitor that straps around your chest under the bra line and transmits your heart rate to a special wrist watch; that way you can check your heart rate instantaneously at any point during your workout.)

If you find it difficult to take your pulse while you're moving or feel unsure you're taking it correctly, you may want to try going by your relative perceived exertion (RPE). This method bases difficulty of exercise on a scale of one to ten, one being very light, easy activity like strolling or leisurely bike riding and ten being near an all-out effort like sprinting up a hill or dashing up stairs two at a time. You should strive to maintain a workout intensity of between five and eight; after you've used the scale for a while, you'll instinctively have a good sense of how hard you are working.

Even using an RPE scale can be confusing, so here's a good rule to keep in mind when you aerobicize: you are working at the correct intensity if you can still carry on a breathless conversation. If you find yourself unable to speak, you're working too hard, and if you can gab at the top of your lungs, pick up the pace!

- *Flexibility:* It's not enough for a muscle to be strong. It must be flexible, too. Flexibility refers to the ability to move your joints through a range of motion. Most fitness experts believe that a good strength-to-flexibility ratio is an important factor for injury prevention, easing muscle soreness after a hard workout, and stress reduction.

You can improve your flexibility by regularly stretching all your major muscle groups. The *Stretching Out* chapter (p. 64) outlines exactly how to do this for your middle muscles. Stretching should be performed at the end of each workout when your muscles are warm and "receptive" to the stretch. Besides, a postworkout stretch is a nice way to cool down your mind: it gives you a chance to relax and spend a few moments reviewing the workout you've just completed.

- *Nutrition:* Many people equate nutrition with dieting, but these two terms are often mutually exclusive. To get the most out of your fitness program, you want to practice healthy eating habits rather than counting calories. Proper nutrition will give you more energy for your workouts and form the building blocks to construct your ideal body.

There are three elemental nutrients: carbohydrates, fats, and proteins. Your body derives most of its energy from carbohydrates which come in two forms, simple and complex. Simple carbs are found in refined and natural sugars such as cookies, candy, and cake, and are easy for your body to break down. They give you a quick burst of energy, but also stimulate the release of large amounts of insulin—which send you crashing back down, craving more energy and more food. Complex carbohydrates, found in grains, cereals, starches (potatoes, pasta, etc.), and vegetables release energy into your system more gradually. They are usually lower in calories and higher in vitamin, mineral, and fiber content. Between 55 and 65 percent of your calorie intake should come from carbohydrates.

Fat is a good source of nutrition and energy, but it's, well, more fattening than either of the other two nutrients. One gram of carbohydrate or protein contains four calories while an equal amount of fat contains nine calories. You should make an effort to keep your fat intake to a minimum—no more than 20 to 25 percent of your daily caloric intake. Dietary fats include oils, butter, marbled meats, nuts, and seeds.

Protein provides the material to build muscle and tissue needed to develop your toned, shapely physique. It's also used as a last-ditch fuel source when carbs and fats aren't available. About 15 to 20 percent of your daily intake should come from protein sources like lean meats, poultry, and fish. Remember, protein doesn't only come from animal sources. Beans, whole grains, and some vegetable sources like potatoes and soy also supply significant amounts of protein without adding a ton of fat to your diet.

Of course, good nutrition is far more complicated than this quick review of the bare basics. Thousands of books have been written to give you a more comprehensive overview on the topic. (Hint: check out the *Buns of Steel Cookbook*.)

Chapter 2

How to Use This Book

Results, Results, Results!

Everyone can create stronger, sexier, sleeker abs by consistently doing the *Abs of Steel* middle-muscle training program. It's a system that's designed to get maximum results in a minimum amount of time. It works because it strengthens and tones all of the muscles that shape your middle, and because it only includes the most effective exercises and most precise techniques. You can customize it to your level and the amount of time you have to devote to training.

Like anything, the *Abs of Steel* system is most effective if you have a thorough understanding of how it works. Read through the information in this chapter before you jump into your middle-muscle training program. You will learn how the book is laid out as well as other important concepts that will help you get the most from your workouts. And there is much more valuable information in the chapters to come!

How The Chapters Are Laid Out

Each of the "exercise" chapters is devoted to one type of exercise, such as isolation moves to strengthen your abdominals, or stretching moves to improve your flexibility. All of the exercise descriptions follow the same general format. Carefully read through the individual exercise descriptions before you start your program. This will help you make each repetition count.

SET-UP:

Pay special attention to these directions. They describe exactly how your body should be positioned at the start of each exercise. The correct starting position is very often the key to getting maximum results.

MOVE:

The photos which accompany each exercise give you a general idea of how to perform the move, but do not rely on them alone. The step by step instruction in this section contains important information to help you do the moves safely and correctly. In *Stretching Out,* pp. 67-74, the Set-up and Move sections are combined.

MIND BODY CONNECTION:

Think of these tips as a link between your body and your brain. They'll help you understand something that may be unfamiliar (an exercise) by relating it to something that's very familiar (like a zipper), or by letting you know precisely what the move should feel like, and where you should feel it.

VARIATIONS:

You can go beyond the basics by adapting each exercise to suit your needs and abilities. We tell you how to change the exercises to make them more challenging or, if need be, how to tone them down.

FORM TIPS:

Here is where we give you the critical do's and don'ts to perfect your exercise form and prevent injury.

The Routines

Once you are familiar with all the exercises, you're ready to begin the routines. They're explained in the *Routines* chapter (p. 76). We've included 5-, 10-, 15- and 20-minute routines for beginner, intermediate, and advanced exercisers as well as split routines which allow you to work different muscle groups on

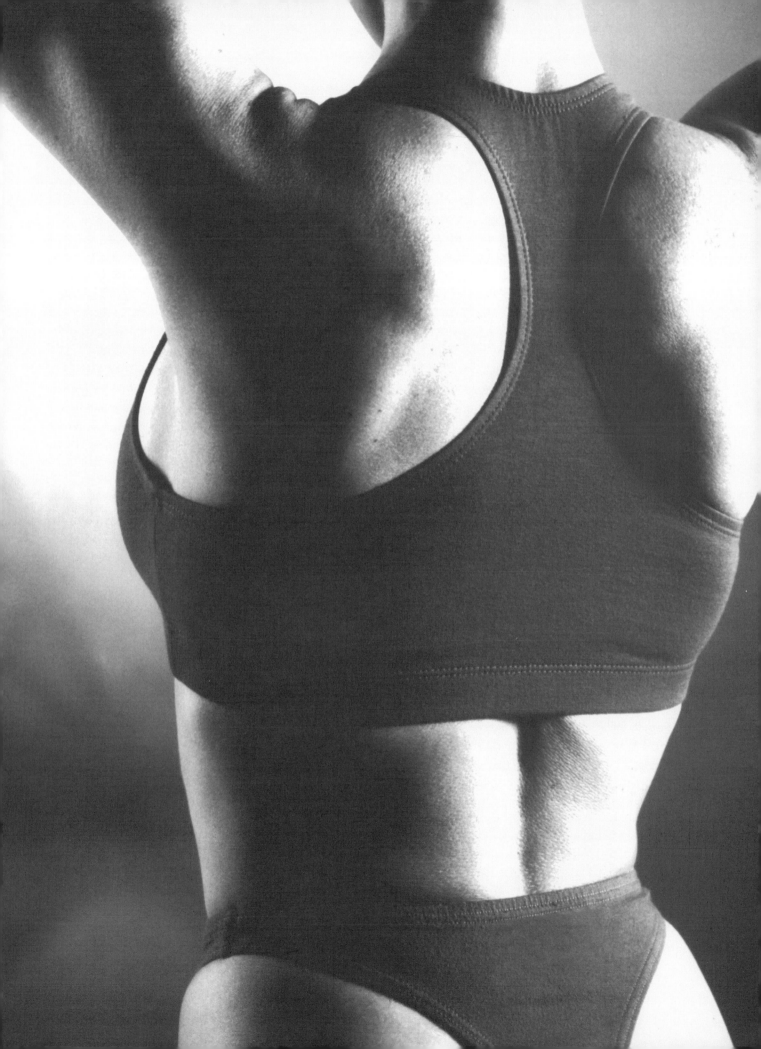

different days. This chapter also explains the number of reps and sets you need to do, the specific variation of the exercise that is appropriate for your level, the amount of rest you should take between sets and workouts, and more.

You should have no problem selecting a routine or group of routines to suit your current fitness needs and time constraints. Once you are comfortable with the exercises and concepts, feel free to experiment and make up your own routines.

The *Breaking Out of Your Routine* chapter (p. 88) offers advice for those with special needs. For instance, if you have a lower-back problem or you are pregnant, flip to this chapter and check out the specially designed routines. There are also tips for making the exercises even more challenging if you are a very advanced exerciser.

The buns exercises and routines are provided separately in a special bonus *Buns of Steel* chapter (p. 94).

Equipment

You don't need a great deal of equipment to get an effective middle-muscle workout. Because the moves are very precise, your body weight should provide enough resistance to work your muscles effectively. All you really need is a cushioned exercise mat or thick bath towel to provide a padded surface for exercises where you lie or sit on the floor, as well as a sturdy chair and a wall. Very advanced exercisers may want to add a 1- to 3-pound dumbbell or an exercise band to some of the exercises.

For the buns exercises, it's a good idea to add extra resistance as you progress in the form of a pair of 3- to 8-pound dumbbells, 1- to 5-pound ankle weights, or an exercise tube or band—depending on the exercise. You'll also need a wall or a chair for some of these exercises.

Avoiding Injury

The exercises in this program are carefully designed to help you avoid injury. As you will see when you read the exercise descriptions, we have been very detailed in describing proper form and explaining exactly how each exercise should feel when you are doing it right. If you follow our directions conscientiously, you may never have to interrupt your training regimen due to injury.

Most injuries are the result of carelessness. If you are performing a move incorrectly or using sloppy form, your body won't feel the effects of the exercises where it should. Worse yet, you may develop a neck or backache. Read the exercise descriptions thoroughly and follow them to the letter. Pay special attention to the *Form Tips.*

Always move slowly through the exercises at a steady, even pace. Never exercise quickly or with abrupt, jerky movements. The object is to feel a contraction or stretch through the working muscles, *not* a jarring sensation through your bones (and teeth)!

You will feel your muscles working hard and pushing to new limits, especially if you haven't done much abdominal work recently. Think of this muscular effort as a mild, *good pain*—working hard but not overdoing it. Once you get used to feeling this good pain, you'll come to enjoy it and understand it as your body's response to the demands **Abs of Steel** training places upon it.

You should *never* experience what we refer to as *bad pain* while doing an exercise or after you've completed your routine. *Bad pain* is the kind you feel in your joints rather than your muscles. If you get a shooting pain through your back, or your neck is throbbing for hours after your workout, perhaps you're working at a level that is too advanced, you're not using correct form, or some of the exercises simply don't work for you. It's important that you learn to differentiate between *good pain* and *bad pain* so that you know when to work through your discomfort and when to back off.

What if, despite precautions, you do injure yourself? Usually, it's best to rest rather than to continue exercising. Better to lay off completely for one week than to do further damage and be forced to lay off for an even longer period of time. If possible, work around an injury by focusing your energies on exercises and routines that don't seem to aggravate the problem. For any problem that seems chronic, it's best to see your doctor.

Muscle Soreness

Some muscle soreness is a normal consequence of proper training, at least initially. You should feel a pleasant sort of muscle fatigue after a good workout—*not* sharp and agonizing pain.

Soreness is caused by internal swelling and microscopic tears in your muscle tissue. When these tiny rips repair, your muscles become stronger, firmer, and shapelier. In fact, it's this constant cycle of tearing down and building back up that helps you achieve maximum tone.

Typically, you'll have some muscle ache immediately following a workout; or you may experience something called *delayed muscle soreness* from 24 to 48 hours following your last exercise session. This may occur after your first few workouts, but if you break your muscles in slowly, soreness should be minimal. As time goes on, and your muscles become used to working out, you shouldn't feel sore after every session unless you are trying a new routine or exercise. In fact, you don't have to feel sore to know that the workout is effective.

However, no workout should make you feel like you've been punched repeatedly in the stomach! If your muscles are so sore that you feel nauseated or you can't stand up straight, you've definitely overdone it. Go easy for the next few days and do as much gentle stretching as the soreness will allow. Whirlpool and massage may temporarily help ease the pain, too. If you follow our routines, work at the proper level, and make impeccable form a priority, soreness shouldn't be a major issue.

Abs of Steel Evaluation

Take this short evaluation to help determine which level of **Abs of Steel** routines you should start with. It will take about five minutes and you will need two, two-inch pieces of masking tape, a mat, a piece of paper and pencil or pen to record your results.

This evaluation is not meant to assess your overall physical condition, health, or well-being, nor is it a medical test: its purpose is to help you determine which level of routines are best suited to your current degree of middle-muscle conditioning.

1. Select the following statement which most closely describes your current abdominal or middle-muscle routine:
   a. I regularly target tone these muscles at least twice a week and have done so for more than three months.
   b. I regularly target tone these muscles at least twice a week and have done so for between one and three months.
   c. I do not regularly target tone these muscles, or have been target toning for less than one month.

2. This test evaluates the flexibility of your hamstrings (backs of your thighs) and lower back. If you have a history of lower-back problems or are currently experiencing discomfort, skip this test and select answer c.

   Remove your shoes and stand with your feet together, knees straight but not "locked." Bend forward and carefully reach for the floor. Choose the statement which most accurately describes the results:
   a. You can touch the floor with little effort and no discomfort in your hamstrings or lower back.
   b. You can just touch your toes. You have no discomfort or only slight discomfort in your hamstrings or lower back.
   c. You can not reach your toes and/or have considerable discomfort in your hamstrings or lower back.

3. This test evaluates lower-back strength; if you have a history of lower-back problems or are currently experiencing discomfort, skip this test and select answer c.

   Lie on your stomach (on your mat) and pull your abs inward. Raise your arms and legs up about one inch off the floor and attempt to hold them in this up position for a slow count of five. Choose the statement that most accurately describes the results:
   a. You had no trouble holding this position for five slow counts, and experienced no lower-back discomfort.
   b. You could just barely hold this position for five counts and/or experienced slight lower-back discomfort.
   c. You could not hold this position for five slow counts and/or you experienced considerable lower-back discomfort.

4. This test evaluates hip flexor (top of thigh) flexibility. Tight hip flexors may limit your range of motion or make it difficult to engage your abdominals during certain exercises.

   Lie on your back (on your mat) and hug one knee gently toward your chest with both hands.

Extend your other leg out straight. Switch legs and repeat. Choose the statement which most accurately describes the results:

    a. Both of your legs, when extended, rest along the floor directly in line with your hip.

    b. One or both of your legs, when extended, rest along the floor to the outside of your hip.

    c. One or both of your extended legs did not touch the floor.

5. This test measures abdominal strength. If you have a history of lower-back problems, or you are currently experiencing discomfort, skip this test and select answer c.

    Place two pieces of masking tape halfway along and at the edge of your mat, one directly behind the other, about two and one-half inches apart. Lie down on your back on the mat with your arms resting on the mat at your sides so that your fingertips are just touching the back edge of the back piece of tape. Bend your knees and place your feet flat on the floor. Curl your head, neck, and shoulder blades upward and, as you do so, slide your palms along the floor until your fingertips touch the front edge of the front piece of tape. Return to the start and repeat for as many reps as you can until you are too tired to continue or you are unable to reach the tape. Choose the statement which most accurately describes the results:

    a. You completed 40 or more repetitions.

    b. You completed 10 to 39 repetitions.

    c. You completed less than 10 repetitions.

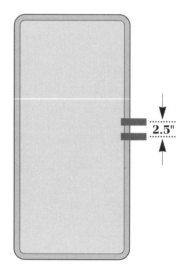

Count up the number of a, b, and c answers you chose. If you have three or more *a* answers, start with the *advanced* routines. If you have three or more *b* answers, start with the *intermediate* routines. If you have three or more *c* answers, start with the *beginner* routines. If you have an equal number of answers of two different letters, start at the lower of the two levels.

Please note: The ***Abs of Steel*** evaluation will give you a general idea of your starting point, but you should begin at the level at which you feel most comfortable.

Chapter 3

Stabilization and Awareness of Your Middle Muscles

Picture a woman you know who has abs *to die for.* Of course she has a sleek, taut tummy, but that's not the only characteristic of someone with great abs. Notice how she carries herself: confidently tall with her stomach naturally pulled inward. Her lower back has a slight curve, but it's not so arched that her belly sticks out. Regardless of whether she has a layer of body fat covering the definition of her muscles, she's firm and flat around the middle.

Fortunately, you don't have to be naturally blessed to have great abs. A large part of sculpting **Abs of Steel** comes from strengthening your middle muscles and perfecting your posture. Even if you never lose an ounce, you can make big improvements by including stabilization and awareness exercises in your **Abs of Steel** routine.

Beyond Crunches

We call the exercises in this chapter stabilization and awareness exercises because they are designed to teach your middle muscles to work together as a group and help you understand how it feels when you use them to support your spine. Rather than isolate each muscle group, these moves work your abs, waist, and lower back simultaneously.

When your middle muscles are strong and working in unison, they pull inward and shape to your spine. You stand taller and your tummy is flatter. You appear to have less flab and more tone—**Abs of Steel**!

But aren't crunches an ideal exercise to help flatten your middle? Yes, but you'll find that doing crunches alone probably won't yield satisfactory results. They isolate one muscle group, your *rectus abdominus* muscle, the long, flat sheet of muscle that runs from the bottom of your rib cage to your pelvis, without using all of your other middle muscles. That's not to say crunches aren't a mandatory part of middle-muscle training, but think about it—how many situations in life call for you to bend forward at the waist twenty times in quick succession?

You are more likely to rely on your *rectus abdominis,* and all the other muscles that form the muscular girdle around your middle, to power many typical, everyday movements like moving a heavy chair across the room, pushing a wheelbarrow through the garden, or carrying a heavy bundle of newspapers to the recycling bin. All of these situations require your middle muscles to work in cooperation, supporting and stabilizing, giving you the strength and leverage to move in a variety of ways. Even if you think you are using your arms and legs exclusively, you depend upon your abs and other middle muscles for balance, power, support, and strength.

After only a few weeks of doing these exercises, you will automatically begin to use your middle muscles properly without much conscious effort. A wonderful transformation will take place in your appearance: your posture will improve, lower-back pain will disappear, allowing you to move with ease and grace, and your abs will be flatter, firmer, and sexier.

How to Use These Exercises

It is often difficult to feel an abdominal exercise in just the right way, even if it's a good exercise and you think you're doing it correctly. Doing your stabilization and awareness exercises at the beginning of your **Abs of Steel** routine can help enhance the effectiveness of

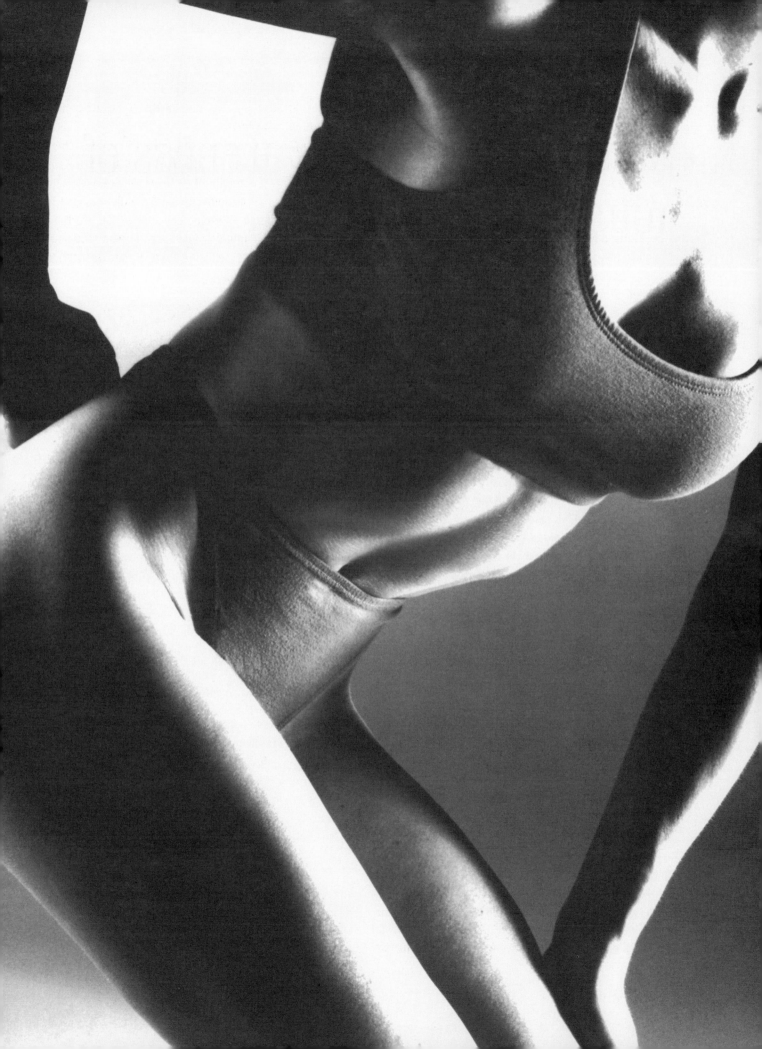

the other types of exercises in the following chapters. They will give you a sense of how your middle muscles should feel when they're properly engaged; consequently, you will feel each repetition in your middle rather than your neck, shoulders, or lower back.

You don't have to do hundreds of repetitions of a stabilization and awareness exercise to get the desired effect—usually 1 to 3 sets of 5 to 12 repetitions done 2 or 3 times a week will be enough. Rest 30 to 90 seconds between each set, long enough to allow your muscles to recover, but not so long that you lose the intensity of your workout.

The key is to do these exercises slowly and carefully, focusing on every point of the movement. Most people will feel a difference after the very first set and see results after just a few weeks of working out. Check out the *Routines* chapter (p. 76) to select the **Abs of Steel** workout most suited to your fitness level and goals.

Before you get started, there is one more thing about these exercises that's important for you to understand: many of them call for you to flatten or round your lower back into the floor. We're not telling you to do this in order to banish the slight, natural curve you have in your lower back. Rather, this is a cue, a physical reminder, to teach you to engage the *erector spinae* and other muscles of the lower back. This is one of the many "focus" techniques you will find throughout this book to help you get the most out of your workout. Your complete **Abs of Steel** routine will actually correct and improve your spinal alignment, because your middle muscles will be stronger and more supportive. You'll look and feel terrific!

Anatomy

The *rectus abdominis* is a long, flat, continuous sheet of muscle which attaches at the bottom of your rib cage and at your pubic bone. Any time you bend from the middle, you are using this muscle. The *transversus abdominis* is located underneath the *rectus.* Although it doesn't initiate any movement, it contracts strongly when you pull your abdominals inward and then exhale. Together these are the two muscles commonly referred to as your abdominals. Whenever you bend or twist to the side, you bring the *internal* and *external obliques* into play. Finally, the *erector spinae* muscles

of your lower back are responsible for lengthening (extending) your spine.

All of these muscles also contract in order to hold your spine in place, or stabilize your torso as you move your body. The aim of the exercises in this chapter is to strengthen and tone your middle muscles in this way. Although you may feel a particular exercise in one particular middle-muscle group more than the others, concentrate on using *all* of them *together* as you do each exercise.

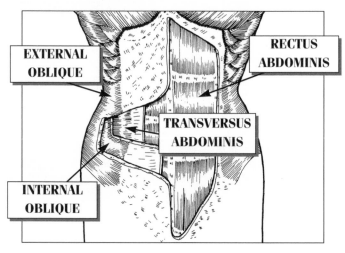

The Exercises in This Chapter

1. Extended Contraction
2. The Slide
3. Stepping
4. Negative Push-Ups
5. Static Crunch
6. Roll-Up
7. The Zipper
8. Pelvic Circles

Extended Contraction

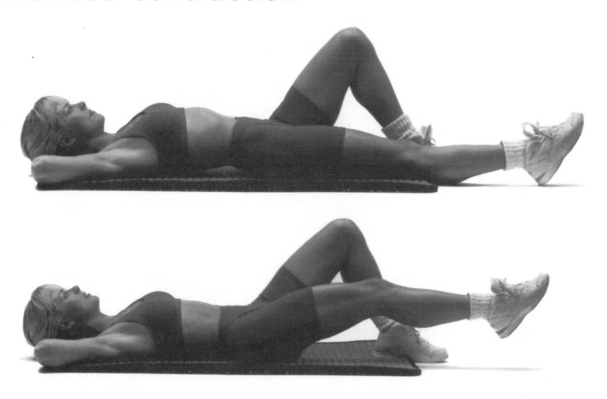

SET-UP:

Lie on your back with your left knee bent, foot flat on the floor, and your right leg extended, toes up, heel into the floor. Place your hands behind your head. Allow your back to arch slightly off the floor so that there is a small space between the small of your back and the floor.

MOVE:

Lift your right leg up off the floor a short way and bend it slightly as you gently squeeze your buns, push your lower back into the floor, and tilt your pelvis upward. Hold for a moment until you feel a strong contraction in your abs. Relax. Do an equal number of reps with both legs.

MIND BODY CONNECTION:

This exercise is similar to the Pelvic Tilt on page 31. However, because your leg is extended and lifted, your muscles, especially your lower-back muscles and *rectus abdominis*, must work harder to initiate the upward tilt of your pelvis. You'll also feel this exercise in your buns.

VARIATIONS:

- To increase the difficulty, lift your leg up without bending it at all.
- To make this exercise less challenging, bend your knee toward your chest as you lift it off the floor until it is even with your bent knee.

FORM TIPS:

- When you relax back to the start, don't overarch your lower back.
- Keep your head, neck, and shoulders relaxed.

The Slide

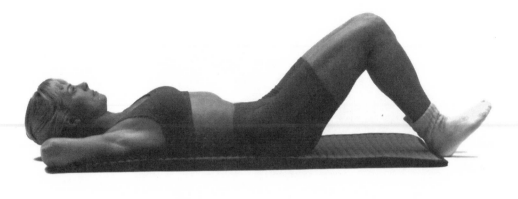

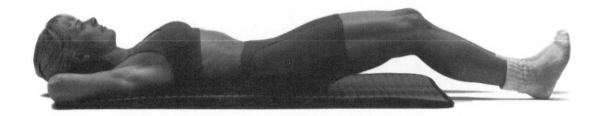

SET-UP:
Remove your shoes. Lie on your back with your knees bent, feet hip-width apart and a comfortable distance from your buns, toes up, heels into the floor. Place your hands behind your head, or wherever they're comfortable. Pull your abs in toward your spine; gently squeeze your buns and tilt your pelvis upward until your back is firmly flattened into the floor.

MOVE:
Slide your heels slowly forward as you gradually straighten your legs. Don't lose the contraction in your abs and don't allow your lower back to pop up off the floor. Once your legs are fully extended, slide your heels back to the start, again taking care not to relax your middle muscles.

MIND BODY CONNECTION:
As you straighten your legs it's harder to keep your back pressed into the floor, so you will have to concentrate on keeping your middle muscles firm and pulled inward. Imagine your entire middle body is weighted down with several sandbags and can't lift off the floor.

VARIATIONS:
• To make this exercise harder, place your heels on two paper plates or a cookie sheet. You'll have to work even harder to slide slowly and with control.
• To make this exercise easier, slide out one heel at a time. Do an equal number of reps with each leg.

FORM TIPS:
• Only slide your legs out as far as you can while still maintaining firm contact with the floor. As you get stronger, gradually increase the range of motion.
• Keep your head, neck, and shoulders relaxed.

Stepping

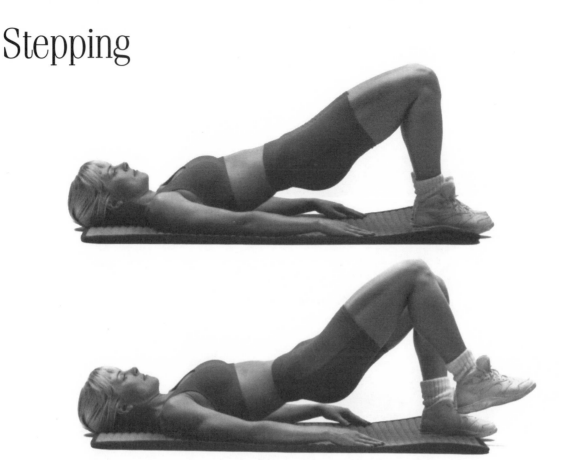

SET-UP:
Lie on your back with your knees bent, feet flat on the floor, hip-width apart and a comfortable distance from your buns, arms down at your sides or wherever they're comfortable. Pull your middle muscles in toward your spine. Keeping your head, neck, and shoulder blades down, lift your back and buns a small way off the floor so there is a straight line from the tops of your shoulders to the tops of your knees.

MOVE:
Hold your set-up position without allowing your spine to sag. Alternate lifting your feet one or two inches off the floor at a moderately slow pace.

MIND BODY CONNECTION:
Use your buns and middle muscles to hold your body still while you step. Done correctly, you'll feel this exercise in your buns as well as your middle muscles.

VARIATIONS:
• For more of a challenge, step faster.

• To make this exercise less challenging, hold the up position for ten seconds without stepping, contracting your middle muscles to maintain a straight spine.

FORM TIPS:
• Keep your steps small.
• Keep your spine in line.

Negative Push-Ups

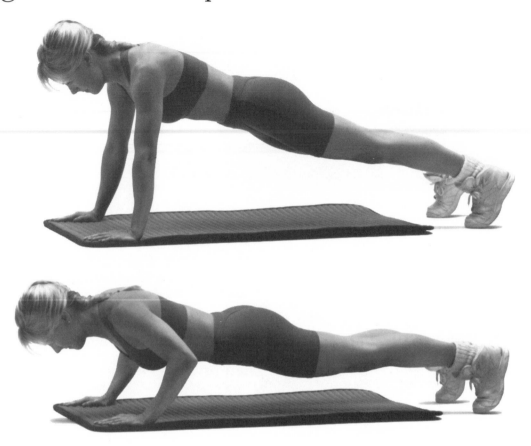

SET-UP:
Lie face down with your toes on the floor, heels upward. With your fingers facing forward and your elbows bent, place your palms on the floor directly underneath your shoulders. Push yourself up by straightening your arms so that you are supporting your weight on your toes and your hands. Pull your middle muscles inward so that your entire spine, including your neck, forms a straight line.

MOVE:
Slowly lower your entire body toward the floor by bending your elbows. Take about five slow counts to reach the floor. As you lower yourself, keep your spine straight by maintaining a strong contraction in your middle muscles.

MIND BODY CONNECTION:
Concentrate on lowering your body as a single unit as if your torso is a flat, unbendable metal sheet.

Although you will feel this exercise in your chest, shoulders, and arms, much of your control and holding power comes from your middle muscles.

VARIATIONS:
To make this exercise more difficult:
- Hold for 3 to 5 slow counts when you have lowered your body halfway to the floor.
- Push up slowly to the start.
- To make this exercise easier, you can bend your knees and lift your lower legs off the floor so that you are balanced on your knees rather than your toes.

FORM TIPS:
- Don't allow your lower back to sag downward.
- Don't arch your neck up, or dip it downward. Tuck your chin slightly and keep your neck in line with your spine.

Static Crunch

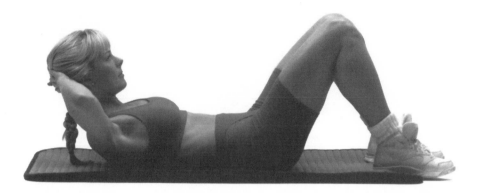

SET-UP:

Lie on your back with your knees bent, feet flat on the floor, hip-width apart and a comfortable distance from your buns. Pull your middle muscles inward. Place your hands behind your head, fingertips touching but not laced together, thumbs behind your ears. Round your elbows outward and tuck your chin a small way toward your chest.

MOVE:

Curl your head, neck, and shoulder blades up and forward off the floor. Hold for five slow counts. Slowly lower to the start.

MIND BODY CONNECTION:

Pretend someone is about to drop a five-pound weight on your stomach and you are tensing up in anticipation.

VARIATIONS:

- If you feel this exercise in your neck, try holding an orange between your chest and chin to learn correct neck alignment.
- Hold for ten slow counts to make this exercise more challenging.

FORM TIPS:

- Don't pull your elbows inward: lift up and hold with your abdominal muscles.

Roll-Up

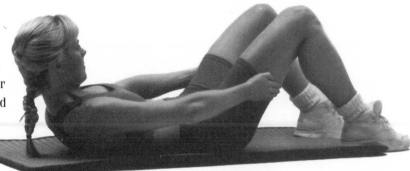

SET-UP:
Lie on your back with your knees bent, feet flat on the floor, hip-width apart and a comfortable distance from your buns, middle muscles pulled in toward your spine. Extend your arms out at your sides and slightly off the floor.

MOVE:
Moving slowly—one vertebra at a time—curl yourself upward. First lift your head off the floor, then your shoulder blades, and, finally, your entire back. Hold onto the back of your thighs for support as soon as you have curled up high enough to comfortably reach them. Use your arm strength for assistance but only as much as is necessary. Continue curling your spine up until your chest touches your knees then sit up tall and hold a moment. Pull your abs in even more, round your back and lower slowly, *with control,* back to the start.

MIND BODY CONNECTION:
Focus on peeling one vertebra at a time off the floor as you move upward, and pasting each of them back in exactly the same spot as you lower.

VARIATIONS:
- To make this harder, hold your hands out to either side of your knees and don't rely on them at all.
- If you find this move too difficult, only do the lowering part. Roll onto your side and push yourself into a seated position.

FORM TIPS:
- Done correctly, this should not cause a strain in your lower back, but if it does, try slowing the move down or try pulling your abs in even more. If it still causes discomfort, skip this exercise and try it again when your middle muscles are stronger.
- Don't throw yourself upward and never use quick or jerky movements.

FOCUS ON FORM:
This exercise is not a full sit-up! The object is to curl yourself off the floor one vertebra at a time rather than lift upward with a straight back.

The Zipper

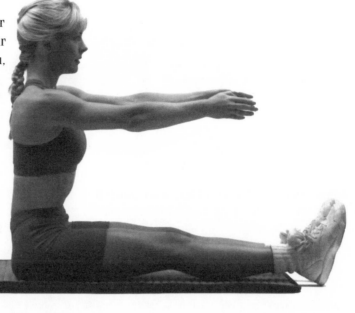

SET-UP:

Sit on the floor, sitting up tall so that your shoulders are aligned directly over your hips. Straighten your legs out in front of you, a few inches apart, feet relaxed. Extend your arms out in front of you at shoulder level. Pull your abs in toward your spine.

MOVE:

Pull your abs inward even more, drop your chin to your chest, and round your back as much as you comfortably can, and reach forward a few inches toward your feet. Hold a moment, and then slowly, one vertebra at a time, straighten up to the start so that you are sitting up very tall. Hold a moment before re-rounding your back and beginning the next rep.

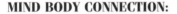

MIND BODY CONNECTION:

Think of the vertebrae in your spine as the teeth of a zipper: as you "zip" upward to sitting, imagine each vertebra stacking directly on top of the one beneath it. As you "unzip" by rounding and reaching forward, imagine each vertebra peeling off the one above it. This exercise should give you a sense of what it is like to sit up straight; the taller you sit and the more you round forward, the more effective it will be. You may also feel a slight stretch through the back of your legs.

VARIATIONS:

- To make this exercise easier, bend your knees slightly.
- To make this exercise harder, place your hands behind your head and hold your elbows out wide.

FORM TIPS:

- Don't force either the rounding or straightening phase.
- Keep your shoulders relaxed and down; don't tighten up your thighs.

Pelvic Circles

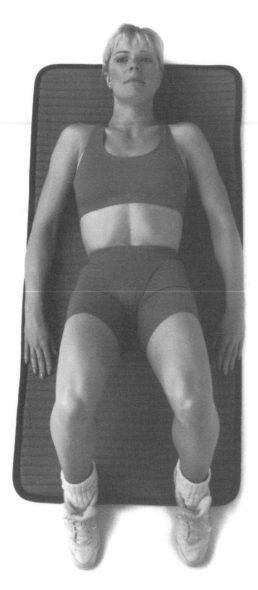

SET-UP:
Lie on your back with your knees bent, feet flat on the floor, hip-width apart, and a comfortable distance from your buns. Rest your arms along your sides. Anchor your back to the floor by pulling all of your middle muscles in toward your spine.

MOVE:
Slowly move your pelvis in a circle: first, pelvic tilt upward by gently squeezing your buns and lifting them 1 to 2 inches off the floor. Next, keeping your hips square to the ceiling, shift your hips slightly to the left. Now slowly relax the pelvic tilt and lower your pelvis to the floor. Then, slide your buns along the floor a small way to the right. While remaining slightly shifted to the right, pelvic tilt upward once again. Finally, bring your hip bones back to center. Do an equal number of clockwise and counterclockwise circles.

MIND BODY CONNECTION:
This is a very small, subtle, continuous movement. Imagine you are drawing a circle the size of a small salad bowl with your tailbone. Each circle should trace

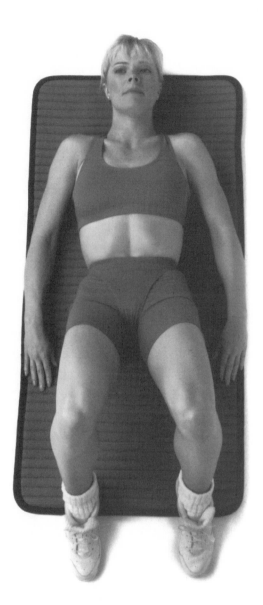 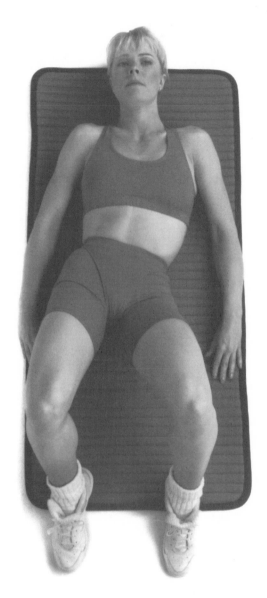

the path of the preceding one. You will also feel a contraction in your buns and hamstrings.

VARIATIONS:

- If you find this exercise too difficult, isolate each movement. For example, first do five pelvis tilts to the left, then do five tilts to the right, and so on.
- To make this exercise harder, trace slightly larger circles.

FORM TIPS:

- Your lower back should remain anchored to the floor throughout.
- Relax your head, neck, and shoulders.

Chapter 4
Your Lower Back

Eighty percent of adult Americans experience lower-back discomfort at some point in their lives. Are you one of them? Discomfort can mean anything from a vague feeling of tightness to sharp, stabbing pains that shoot through your back. You may feel an occasional twinge or endure constant, chronic pain.

Just because your lower back hurts, it doesn't mean there's something drastically wrong with your spine. Your pain is more likely to be caused by some sort of muscular imbalance.

Imagine walking around all day with a ten-pound weight loosely strapped to your stomach. You'd have to compensate for this extra weight by arching your lower back, locking your knees, and slouching forward at the neck, shoulders, and hips. After a while, your back would begin to ache from the stress and strain of hauling around this excess load.

Well, that's essentially what it's like when you're carrying a little extra body fat around your middle and your muscles aren't strong enough to bear the burden. That's why it's so important to maintain a healthy amount of body fat and keep your middle muscles strong and in top condition. The exercises in the *Your Abdominals* chapter (p. 40) strengthen your abdominal muscles, and that's a great start. However, it's just as important to strengthen and tone the muscles opposite them, your lower-back muscles, as well.

Tight, weak lower-back muscles, along with out-of-shape abdominal and oblique muscles, are often the root of lower-back problems. Doctors once believed painkillers or surgery was the best way to manage lower-back pain, but increasingly, health and medical experts recommend doing exercises like the ones in this chapter for effective, lasting relief. Like any other muscle in your body, your lower-back muscles respond to regular exercise by growing stronger and more supple. Of course, if you have a history of severe back problems, you should always check with your doctor before beginning this or any exercise program.

Some of the exercises in this chapter work by strengthening your back extensor muscles, the muscles along the length of your lower spine. Strong extensor muscles work in tandem with your abdominals and obliques to support your lower spine and keep it injury free. Other exercises in the chapter lengthen and stretch your back extensors—good flexibility can also protect against injury.

Perhaps you never thought of it this way, but banishing lower-back pain will not only make you feel better, it will also improve your appearance. When your lower back is stronger and more flexible, you are able to stand up straighter, sit up taller in your chair, and move with the grace of a dancer. Without shedding an ounce, you'll immediately appear sleeker, taller, trimmer.

But what if you are one of the lucky ones who has never had so much as a twinge of lower-back pain? You may never have thought to include lower-back exercises in your **Abs of Steel** training, because you don't have problems and you don't face this part of your body in the mirror every day. However, working your lower-back muscles will definitely help firm up your middle, and whittle down your waist measurement! Include the exercises in this chapter as part of your **Abs of Steel** middle-muscle training program to help firm and shape your lower-back area. By giving sagging back muscles a lift, you reduce that spare tire effect around your middle, allowing your flat, toned tummy to grab the spotlight.

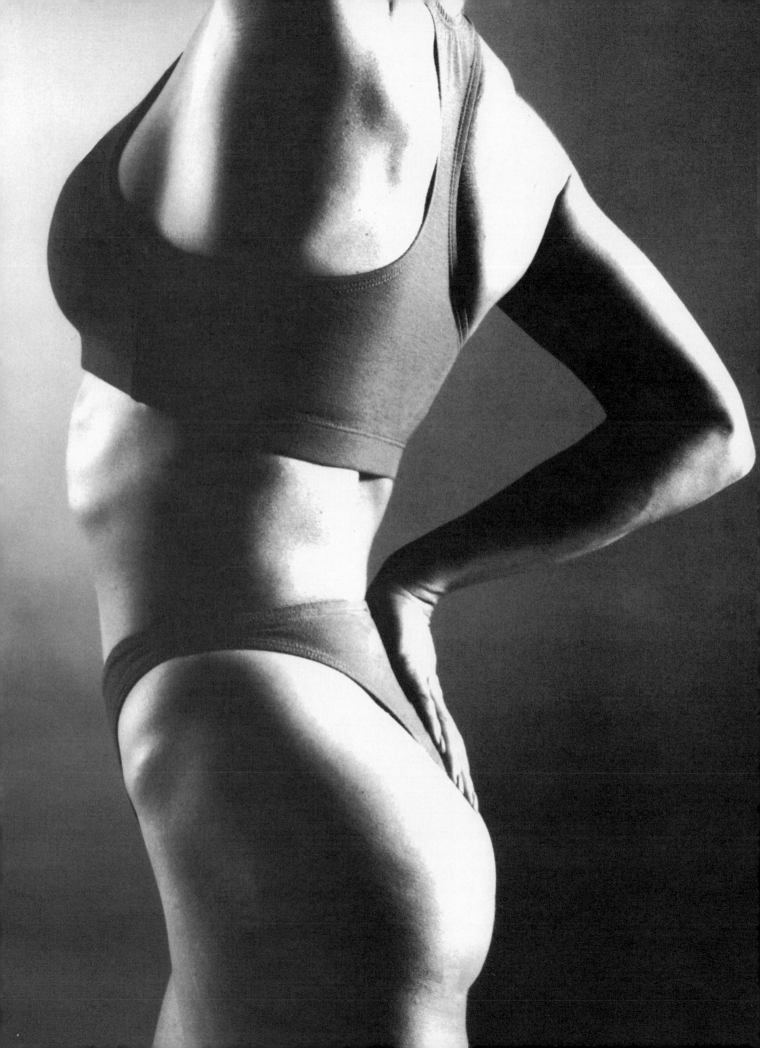

Keep in mind that back strength and flexibility are highly individual things. There are exercises in this chapter like Press-Ups which call for you to lift your head, shoulders, and chest off the floor while lying on your stomach. You may be able to raise your entire chest off the floor, but more likely, you'll only be able to lift up a few inches. Whatever your level and ability, move through the range of motion that's comfortable for you. Never force anything to the point of pain.

Even if you aren't very strong or supple to begin with, you will still benefit from doing these exercises. Lower-back muscles tend to increase in strength and flexibility very quickly. You'll see increased tone and better posture in just a few short weeks if you include the exercises in this chapter in your **Abs of Steel** training program.

How To Use These Exercises

Doing your lower-back exercises after your stabilization and awareness exercises and before the rest of your middle-muscle training further warms up your lower-back muscles and prepares them to handle the rest of your abdominal workout without undue stress and strain. Include at least one strengthening and one stretching exercise for your lower back once you begin doing the intermediate and advanced routines of more than five minutes. Do only the stretches if you are just starting out or you are prone to persistent back problems. Once your lower back becomes more flexible, you can add the strengthening exercises. We'll note in the *Mind Body Connection* section what the specific purpose of each exercise is and where you should feel it most.

The number of sets and repetitions you will need to do varies from exercise to exercise. In general, you should include 2 to 3 sets of 8 to 12 repetitions, 2 to 3 times a week, of lower-back training in your **Abs of Steel** routine. Rest 30 to 90 seconds between each set; long enough to allow your muscles to recover, but not so long that you lose the intensity of your workout.

Check out the *Routines* chapter (p. 76) for the exact number of reps and sets appropriate for your fitness level. If your lower back is stiff and tight, you may feel looser and more limber after just one workout. Most people will see visible improvements in just a few weeks.

Anatomy

The *erector spinae* are a group of muscles that attach to your lower spine and are your main "back extensor" muscles. Any time you lean backward or lift your head, shoulders, and chest off the floor while lying on your stomach, you are using your *erector spinae* and other back extensor muscles.

Not all the exercises in this chapter work your lower-back muscles by asking them to contract in order to strengthen them. The Pelvic Tilt, for example, is a move designed to lengthen and stretch your back extensors. The purpose of each exercise is noted in its description.

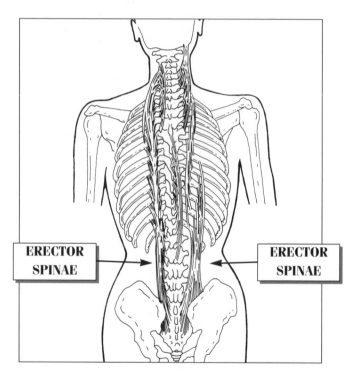

The Exercises in This Chapter

1. Pelvic Tilt
2. Chair Tilt
3. The Fulcrum
4. Cat-Cow
5. Press-Up
6. Back Sweep
7. Swimming
8. The Ball

Pelvic Tilt

SET-UP:

Lie on your back with your knees bent, feet flat on the floor, hip-width apart and a comfortable distance from your buns. Place one hand on your stomach and one hand, palm down, directly underneath the small of your back. Gently press your back into your hand and pull your abdominals in toward your spine so that your entire lower back is firmly anchored to the floor.

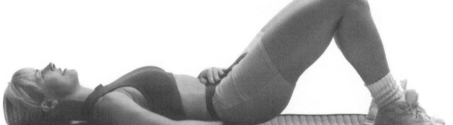

MOVE:

Keeping your entire back anchored, gently squeeze your buns together and tilt your hips up until your buns curl 1 or 2 inches off the floor. Hold a moment and slowly lower to the start. (Note: Remember that anchoring means pulling your abdominals inward and firmly pressing your lower back into the floor.)

MIND BODY CONNECTION:

Use the hand on your stomach to remind you not to push your abdominals outward; use the pressure of your body on your other hand to remind you not to lose contact between your back and the floor or your hand, even when you lower to the start. You will feel your lower back lengthen and relax as you tilt upward; you'll also feel a contraction in your buns, the back of your thighs, and your abs.

VARIATIONS:

• When you feel sure you're doing this exercise correctly, place your hands anywhere they're comfortable (behind your head or on the floor at your sides).

FORM TIPS:

• Keep your head, neck, and shoulders relaxed.
• Don't lift your lower back off the floor as you tilt your pelvis upward, and don't arch it off the floor when you lower to the start.

FOCUS ON FORM:

Don't allow your lower back to lift up off the floor! Firmly anchor your spine by pulling your abs inward and pressing your back into the floor.

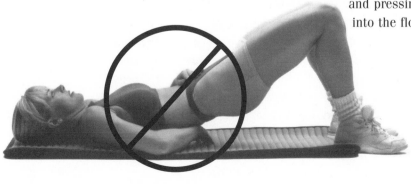

Chair Tilt

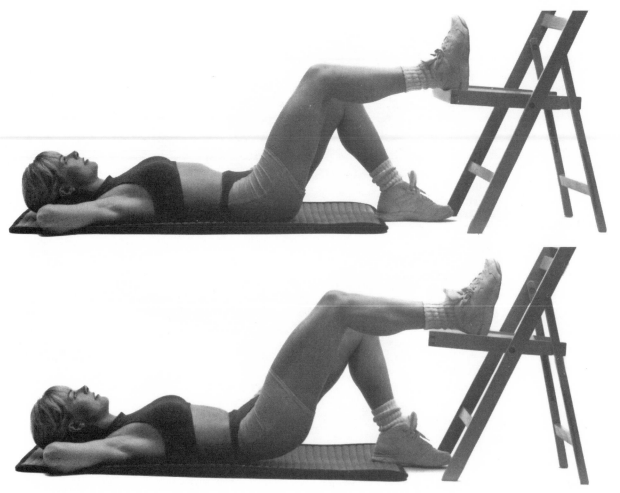

SET-UP:
Lie on your back about half-a-leg's length away from a sturdy chair. Bend your left knee so that your foot is flat on the floor a comfortable distance from your buns. Rest your right heel up on the seat of the chair. Gently press your back into the floor and pull your abdominals in toward your spine.

MOVE:
Keeping your entire back firmly anchored to the floor, gently squeeze your buns together and tilt your hips up until your buns curl 1 or 2 inches off the floor. Hold a moment and slowly lower to the start. Switch legs and do an equal number of reps.

MIND BODY CONNECTION:
Press your heel downward into the chair as a reminder to tilt your pelvis and contract your middle muscles.

You'll feel your lower back lengthen as you tilt upward; you'll also feel a strong contraction in your buns, back of thighs, and abdominals.

VARIATIONS:
• For more of a challenge, place both feet up on the chair and tilt upward.
• If you find this exercise too difficult, place your foot on a lower object such as a step or a thick book.

FORM TIPS:
• Your hips should remain level throughout the movement.
• Your lower back should remain firmly anchored to the floor throughout the exercise.
• Don't use a very tall chair for this exercise; a sturdy, non-rolling office or kitchen chair is ideal.

The Fulcrum

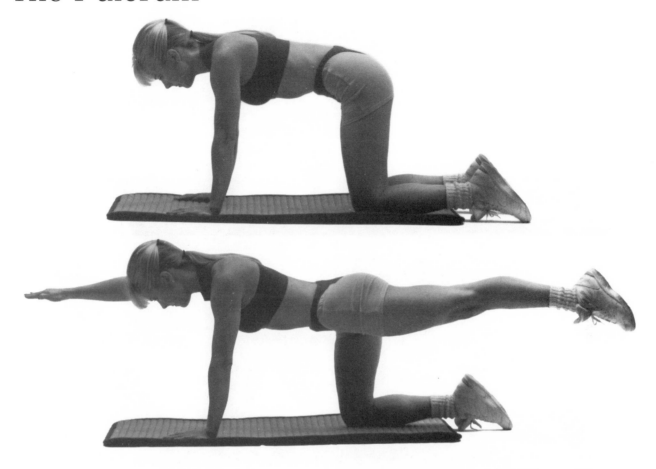

SET-UP:
Kneel on your hands and knees so that your arms and legs form a box. Your hands should be directly underneath your shoulders, knees directly underneath your hips. Tuck your chin a little toward your chest so that your entire spine, including your neck, is aligned. Pull your abs inward and don't allow your lower back to sag.

MOVE:
Extend your right arm straight in front of you at shoulder level, and your left leg directly behind you at hip level. Concentrate on pushing out your arm and leg as much as possible until you feel a stretching and lengthening through all of your back. Hold for a slow count of five and return to the start. Do an equal number of reps using your left arm and right leg.

MIND BODY CONNECTION:
Pretend you are trying to touch something just out of

reach of your fingertips and toes. You'll feel a stretch through the length of your spine, and your spine will align as you reach.

VARIATIONS:
- To make this exercise harder, do it while lying on your stomach. Lengthen your arm and leg as you hold them a few inches off the floor; don't reach up any higher than shoulder and hip height.
- To make this exercise easier, lift your arm up first, placing your hand back on the floor before you lift up your leg.

FORM TIPS:
- Keeping your abs pulled inward will increase the stretch.
- Don't lift your arm or leg above shoulder or hip height.

Cat-Cow

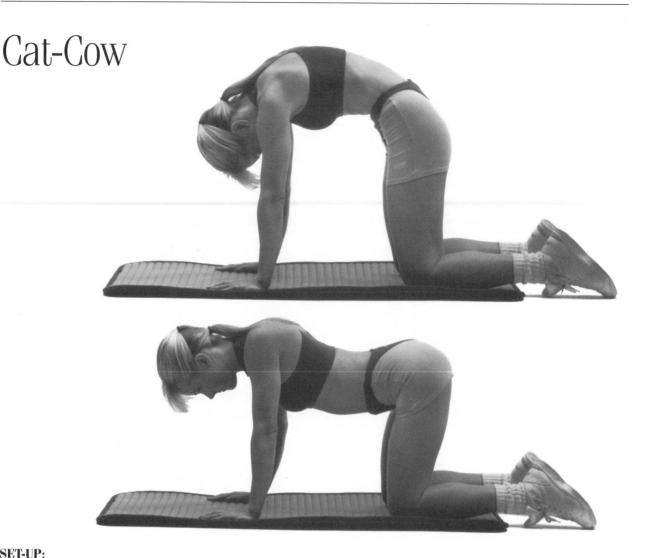

SET-UP:

Kneel on your hands and knees so that your arms and legs form a box. Your hands are directly underneath your shoulders, knees directly underneath your hips. Align your spine by tucking your chin a small way toward your chest and pulling your abs inward.

MOVE:

Slowly arch your back and allow your belly to sag toward the floor. Hold until you feel a stretch through your abdominals, and then pull your abs way up into your rib cage so that you arch upward and feel a stretch through the entire length of your back. Move up and down through these two positions continuously.

MIND BODY CONNECTION:

As you arch downward, think of the swayback of a cow; as you arch upward, think of a frightened cat. Arch in each direction only as much as you feel comfortable doing. You'll feel your back extensors contract as you arch downward and stretch as you arch upward.

VARIATIONS:

- To make this move more challenging, hold a moment in the center of the movement by pulling your abs inward and lengthening your spine.
- If you feel lower-back discomfort on the downward arch, only do the upward half of the exercise; if you feel the discomfort on the upward arch, discontinue the downward arch.

FORM TIPS:

- Keep your neck aligned with the rest of your spine; don't tilt your neck up and down as you go through the movement.
- Keep your arms and legs still throughout the movement.
- Keep your shoulders and neck relaxed.

Press-Up

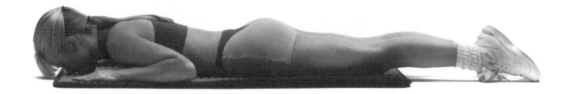

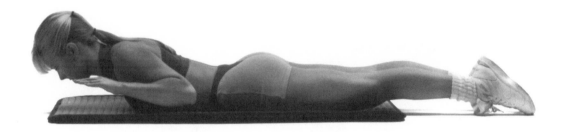

SET-UP:

Lie on your stomach with your forehead on the floor, your hands directly underneath your shoulders, elbows at your sides, and your legs together and extended straight out behind you. Pull your abs inward as if you are trying to create a small space between your stomach and the floor.

MOVE:

Keeping your feet on the floor, squeeze your buns and thighs together as you lift your head, shoulders, and chest up off the floor. Don't use your hands to help push you higher. Hold a moment, and return to the start.

MIND BODY CONNECTION:

When you are in the pressed-up position, lift your hands a small way off the floor to make sure you're not using them to assist you. You'll feel a strong pull through your back extensors as you lift upward. You'll also feel this exercise in your buns and inner thighs.

VARIATIONS:

- If your lower back is strong enough to do so, and you feel you can arch up higher, you may use your hands to assist you upward another inch.
- If this exercise causes discomfort in your lower back, try pressing up by placing your forearms on the floor and making fists with your hands. If this still feels uncomfortable, skip this exercise and try it when your lower back is stronger (after about a month of working out).

FORM TIPS:

- Don't force the lifting phase.
- Keep your shoulders relaxed and down and your neck in line with your spine.

Back Sweep

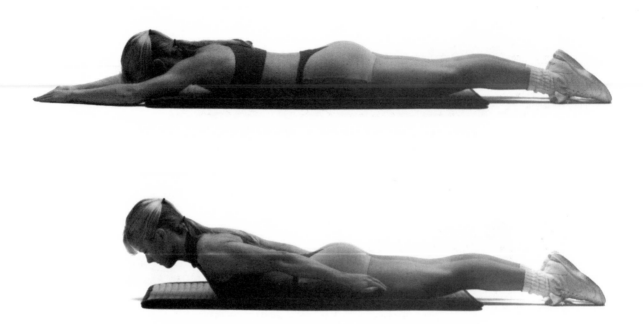

SET-UP:

Lie on your stomach with your forehead on the floor. Extend your arms out in front of you, palms downward, and extend your legs straight out behind you. Pull your abs inward as if you are trying to create a small space between your stomach and the floor.

MOVE:

Squeeze your buns and thighs together as you lift your arms, head, shoulders, and chest off the floor. Then, keeping your arms as straight as you can, sweep them back in a wide arc until they're down along your sides. Your palms should remain facing downward throughout the move. Sweep your arms back to the front and lower your body to the start before beginning the next repetition.

MIND BODY CONNECTION:

Move your arms "with resistance" by pretending you are sweeping them through the water, just below the surface. You will feel a strong pull through your back extensors as you lift and hold the up position. This exercise is terrific for improving upper body posture as well as strengthening your buns and inner thighs.

VARIATIONS:

- For more of a challenge, continue the sweep, bringing your hands together behind your back or as close together as your shoulder flexibility will allow.
- If you find this exercise too challenging:
  - Try bending your elbows a few inches.
  - Try sweeping your arms until they are out to the side at shoulder level.
- If the exercise is still too difficult, sweep your arms without raising your head, shoulders, and chest off the floor.

FORM TIPS:

- Lengthen your neck by tucking your chin toward your chest and keep your shoulders relaxed.
- To protect your lower back, maintain the squeeze in your buns and thighs, especially as you lift and hold in the up position.

Swimming

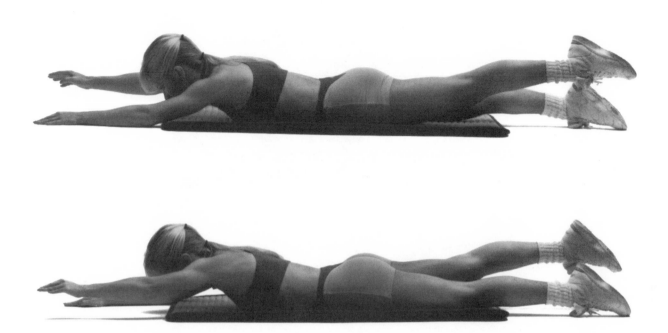

SET-UP:

Lie on your stomach with your forehead on the floor, chin tucked a small way toward your chest. Extend your arms out in front of you, palms downward, and your legs straight out behind you. Lift your right arm and left leg up about an inch off the floor. Lift your head and shoulders off the floor. Pull your abs inward.

MOVE:

Lower your right arm and left leg to the floor as you simultaneously bring your left arm and right leg up to the same height. Continuously alternate at a moderate pace until you've completed all reps.

MIND BODY CONNECTION:

Pretend you're "fluttering" through the water, making a steady, foaming splash with your arms and legs.

VARIATIONS:

- Once you learn the coordination of this exercise, move your arms and legs faster. You'll feel a continuous contraction in your lower back as you complete all swimming reps.
- To make this exercise more difficult, lift your arms and legs slightly above shoulder and hip height.
- To make this exercise easier, keep your forehead, shoulders, and chest on the floor while you flutter only your arms.

FORM TIPS:

- Your head and shoulders should remain lifted until you've completed all reps.
- Keep your shoulders relaxed.

The Ball

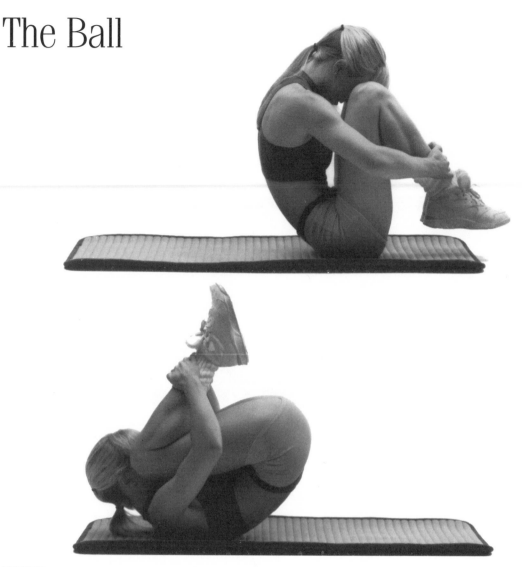

SET-UP:

Sit on the floor and hug your knees to your chest. Keep your shoulders down and relaxed and abs pulled inward toward your spine so that your back is rounded. Open your knees slightly and drop your chin to your chest so that your head is between your knees. Point your toes and balance on your tailbone so that your feet are just off the floor.

MOVE:

Pull your abs even further inward until you roll backward. Roll until your shoulder blades contact the floor and then, without using momentum, roll upward into the balanced position.

MIND BODY CONNECTION:

This exercise will massage, align, and increase the flexibility of your lower back. Make sure you roll through the center of your spine both on the way up and the way down. Done correctly, you will also feel a strong contraction in your abs as you do this exercise.

VARIATIONS:

- You may find it challenging enough to simply find and hold the balanced position.
- To make this exercise more difficult, hold briefly in the rolled back position before returning to the start.

FORM TIPS:

- Concentrate on initiating the rolling with your ab muscles rather than with momentum or by kicking your legs up.
- Don't roll back any farther than your shoulder blades.
- Keep your body in as compact a ball as possible.

Chapter 5

Your Abdominals

A perfect stomach is the crowning jewel of any physique. It draws more attention to you than perhaps any other body part. If your stomach (that's how most people refer to their abdominal muscles) is flabby and out of shape, *you* look out of shape. But if your tummy is tightly toned, you look like you are in peak condition. And there's certainly nothing sexier than a flat, muscular midriff peeking through a short shirt or bikini.

Many exercisers strive for sculpted abs, but, because they use the wrong methods, they often fall short of their goal. Doing the **Abs of Steel** exercises in this chapter is a great way to tone and define your abdominals. Anyone who faithfully includes them in their middle-muscle training routine can sculpt a sleeker, slimmer stomach.

Keep in mind that you can't "spot reduce" your stomach (or any other area of your body for that matter). In other words, all the abdominal exercises in the world won't magically melt away tummy fat. The best way to lose unwanted, excess pounds around your middle, or anywhere else on your body, is by doing at least twenty minutes of aerobic exercise three to five times a week and by following a healthy, low-fat eating plan.

However, you can—and certainly should—target tone your abdominal muscles. Even if you've got an extra layer of fat covering them, you'll still get noticeable results by doing the exercises in this chapter. They'll help pull in and chisel your stomach area, causing it to get smaller and flatter.

All of these abdominal exercises are variations on what are often called "stomach crunches" or "abdominal curl-ups." Crunches have long been the corner-stone of virtually all middle-muscle training programs, and for a good reason. They really work. Crunches involve bending, or flexing, your spine by moving your upper body, lower body, or both at the same time, a small way toward your middle. This movement causes an intense shortening and contraction of the muscles that run the length of your torso.

Done precisely and on a regular basis, crunches are the most effective way to flatten your stomach, whether or not you lose body fat. They trim inches from your waist by firming abdominal muscles and lifting them upward and inward toward your spine.

Middle-Muscle Myths

A common mistake with crunch type exercises is the "more is better" mentality. If doing a few reps of a particular exercise is good, the reasoning goes, then doing hundreds must be even better.

On the contrary. If you can do hundreds of repetitions of a move, it's not intense or precise enough to produce changes in tone or strength of the muscle. One to three sets of fifteen to twenty reps of ab crunches in conjunction with the rest of your **Abs of Steel** training program will give you excellent results. Most people see big improvements after about a month. If you find you can easily do more than twenty reps of an exercise, there's a good chance you're doing something wrong. Slow down and review your form. Are you moving too quickly and relying on momentum to swing you through the movement? Are you helping yourself upward by pulling on your neck with your hands? Are you allowing your abs to protrude outward? Are you holding your breath? If you honestly feel you've corrected all of these common form mistakes,

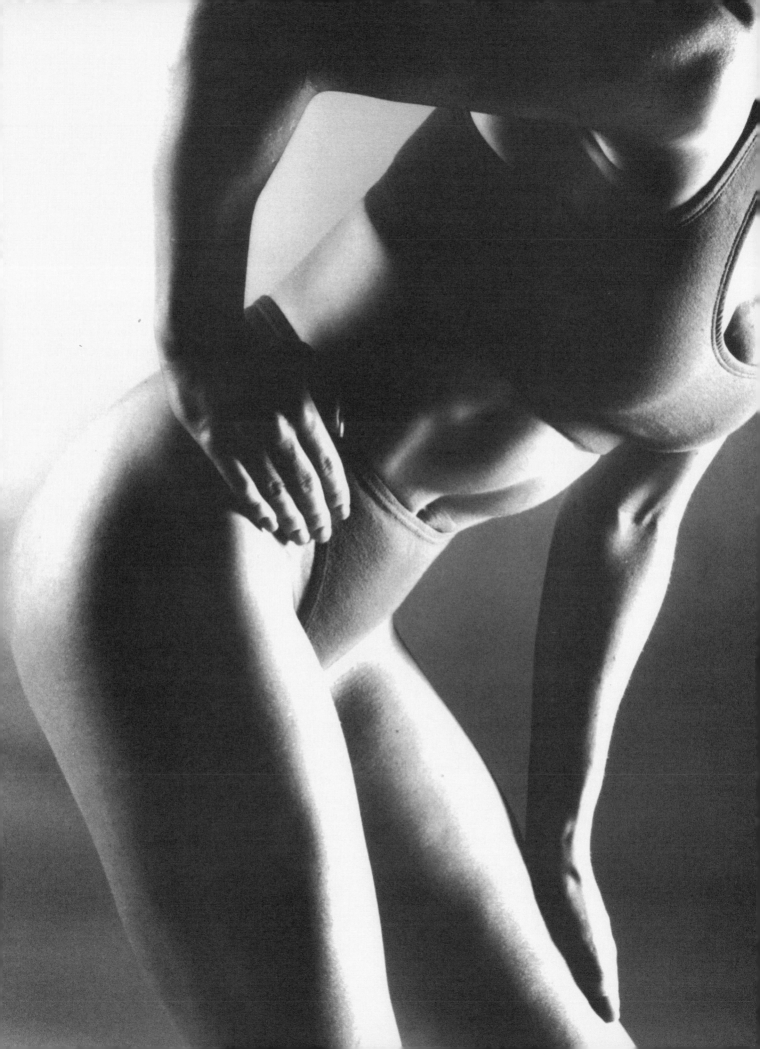

and the exercise *still* seems too easy, it's time to move onto the more difficult variations.

Another common "more is better" misconception is that full sit-ups are better than crunches because you move your body through a greater range of motion. In actuality, your abdominals are only active in the first thirty degrees of a forward bend—which is precisely how far an abdominal crunch will take you—lifting up any higher than that will place a great deal of strain on your lower back. Moreover, if you lock your feet into place by jamming them under your bed or a couch, you essentially deactivate your abdominal muscles and place a greater demand on the *ilio psoas*, your main hip flexor muscle. In fact, an overworked *ilio psoas* will tug downward on your lower vertebrae, causing an extreme arch of your lower back, making your tummy stick out, wrecking your posture and, quite often, causing lower-back pain. Doing abdominal crunches correctly helps balance your ab-to-psoas strength ratio so your stomach is flatter, your posture is better, and lower-back pain is eliminated.

Having said all this, you may notice that the roll-up, an exercise in the *Stabilization and Awareness* chapter (p. 16), calls for you to lift your entire back off the floor. It is important to understand the difference between this exercise and a "full sit-up." The purpose of the roll-up is to increase the mobility of your spine and to hold all of your middle muscles inward as you move through a complete range of motion. Also, you don't simply lift and lower your back off the floor as you would when you do a "full sit-up." You slowly roll your spine up and down off the floor one vertebra at a time.

How To Use These Exercises

Doing your abdominal exercises after the stabilization and awareness and lower-back exercises in the preceding chapters ensures that all of your middle muscles are properly warmed up and prepared for the task of flexing your spine off the floor. You should include at least one of the exercises in this chapter in any *Abs of Steel* routine you do. As you do the abdominal exercises, try to concentrate on the muscle movement just below your chest and just above your hips. You'll feel a strong pull, or contraction, at different points along the abdominal wall, depending upon which exercise you are doing.

The number of sets and repetitions you will do varies from exercise to exercise but in general, you should include 1 to 3 sets of 12 to 20 repetitions, 2 or 3 times a week, of abdominal muscle training in your *Abs of Steel* routine. Rest 30 to 90 seconds between each set; long enough to allow your muscles to recover, but not so long that you lose the intensity of your workout.

Check out the *Routines* chapter (p. 76) for the exact number of reps, sets, and exercises we recommend for your fitness level. As we've said, most people will see visible improvements in as little as one month of working out.

Anatomy

The *transversus abdominis* is the deepest of all your abdominal muscles. Its fibers run perpendicular to your spine. You use this muscle whenever you exhale forcefully, cough, or sneeze. That's why pulling your abs inward and exhaling strongly through your mouth during the effort phase of any exercise in this book will tighten and tone your *transversus abdominis*. However, since you can't isolate this muscle through movement of your spine, the most effective way to work it is by using proper breathing and form during exercise. This will strengthen your other middle muscles, especially the exercises in this chapter and the *Stabilization and Awareness* chapter (p. 16).

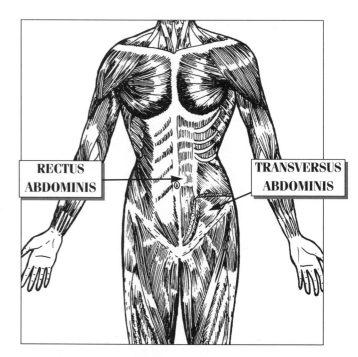

RECTUS ABDOMINIS

TRANSVERSUS ABDOMINIS

On top of the *transversus abdominis* lies your *rectus abdominis*. This is a wide, flat sheet of muscle that runs the vertical length of your torso, attaching at the top to your lower ribs and sternum and to your pelvis at the bottom. It works in conjunction with your oblique muscles to flex; in other words, to bend your spine forward. The *rectus* is also the muscle most commonly referred to as your "abdominals."

Although, technically speaking, your *rectus* is one long continuous muscle, you'll do exercises for both the upper and lower half. Crunch-type exercises where you lift your head, neck, and shoulders off the floor emphasize the upper *rectus*. Exercises where you lift your tailbone off the floor or bring your knees closer to your chest emphasize the lower *rectus*.

The Exercises in This Chapter

1. Basic Crunch
2. Crunch and Curl
3. Single Straight Leg Crunch
4. Crunch and Point
5. Four-Count Crunch
6. Reach and Crunch
7. Double Crunch
8. Reverse Crunch

Basic Crunch

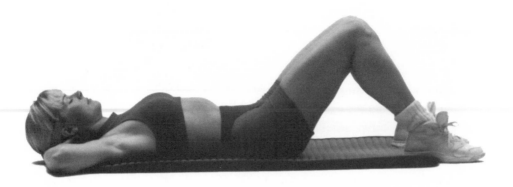

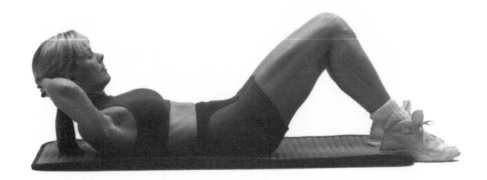

SET-UP:

Lie on your back with your knees bent and your feet flat on the floor, hip-width apart and a comfortable distance from your buns. Place your hands behind your head so that your thumbs are behind your ears. *Don't lace your fingers together.* Hold your elbows out wide and tuck your chin slightly toward your chest. Round your lower back into the floor by gently pulling your abdominals in toward your spine and tilting your pelvis upward.

MOVE:

Curl up and forward so that your head, neck, and shoulder blades lift off the floor. Hold for a moment at the top of the movement then lower slowly to the start.

MIND BODY CONNECTION:

During the upward phase, imagine someone is firmly pressing on the center of your stomach, and you need to tense up your abs in order to resist the pressure. You'll feel tension just below your rib cage as you curl

upward; this tension will spread through the entire abdominal area as you near completion of the set.

VARIATIONS:

- If this move is too difficult, fold your arms across your chest, palms down, and tuck your chin so that it rests on your hands.
- For more of a challenge, "pulse" 5 to 10 times at the top of the movement by moving slightly up and down.

FORM TIPS:

- Keep your lower back firmly on the floor throughout the movement.
- To keep your neck properly aligned, leave some space between your chin and chest as if you're holding an orange there.
- Don't lift upward by pulling on your neck with your hands.

Crunch and Curl

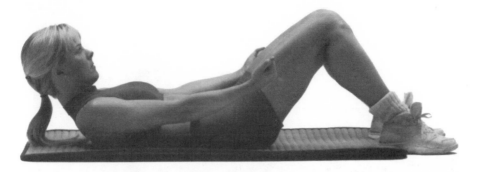

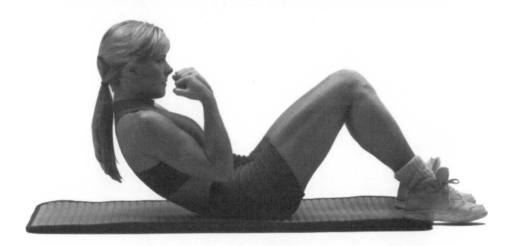

SET-UP:

Lie on your back, knees bent, your feet on the floor hip-width apart and a comfortable distance from your buns. Extend your arms straight out along the floor at your sides. With your palms up, curl your hands into fists. Pull your abs inward and flatten your back into the floor.

MOVE:

Curl your head, neck, and shoulder blades off the floor while at the same time you bend your elbows and curl your fists toward your shoulders. Hold a moment at the top of the movement before lowering to the start.

MIND BODY CONNECTION:

Curling your arms will not only tone your biceps (front of your upper arms) it will also remind you to tighten your abdominal muscles every time you crunch upward.

VARIATIONS:

- For more of a challenge, stay at the top of the movement and "pulse" both your abs and arms 5 to 10 times before lowering back to the start.
- To make this exercise less challenging, place one hand behind your head and do biceps curls with one arm at a time. Do an equal number of reps with both arms.

FORM TIPS:

- Lengthen your neck by tucking your chin a small ways toward your chest; keep your shoulders relaxed.

Single Straight Leg Crunch

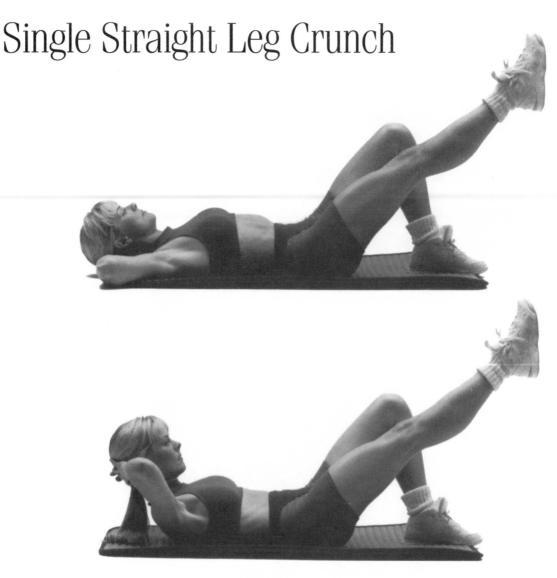

SET-UP:

Lie on your back with your left knee bent, foot flat on the floor and a comfortable distance from your buns. Your right leg should be straight and held up off the floor high enough so you can just see your gently pointed toes. Place your hands behind your head, fingertips touching but not laced together, thumbs behind your ears. Hold your elbows outward. Pull your abs inward.

MOVE:

Curl up and forward so that your head, neck, and shoulder blades lift off the floor. Hold for a moment at the top of the movement then slowly lower to the start. Switch legs and do an equal number of reps.

MIND BODY CONNECTION:

Focus your eyes on the toe of your outstretched leg; move toward it as you lift upward.

VARIATIONS:

• Doing this exercise with both legs extended makes it more challenging.
• Bending your outstretched leg slightly makes this exercise easier.

FORM TIPS:

• Keep your shoulders down and relaxed as you do this movement.
• Keep your outstretched leg still as you move through the exercise.
• Avoid overarching your lower back.

Crunch and Point

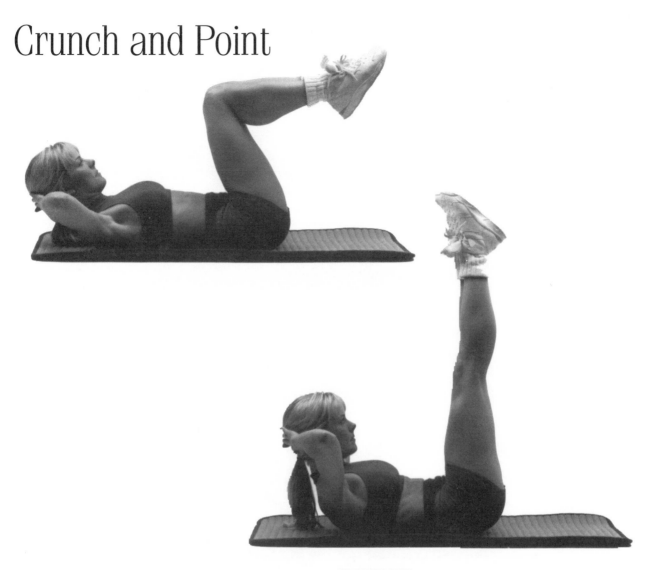

SET-UP:
Lie on your back with your hands behind your head, fingertips touching, thumbs behind your ears. Bend your knees and lift your legs so that your knees are directly over your hips and your lower legs are parallel to the floor. Pull your abs inward and press your back into the floor.

MOVE:
Curl your head, neck, and shoulders up off the floor while at the same time straightening your legs upward. Hold for a moment at the top of the movement and return to the starting position.

MIND BODY CONNECTION:
Pretend you have strings attached to your shoulders and ankles that are all being pulled upward at the same time.

VARIATIONS:
• To make this exercise more difficult, begin with your arms extended out on the floor at your sides, palms facing inward. As you curl upward, reach for your knees.
• To make this exercise easier, only extend your legs halfway upward.

FORM TIPS:
• Your elbows should remain in the same position throughout the movement so you don't pull upward on your neck.

Four-Count Crunch

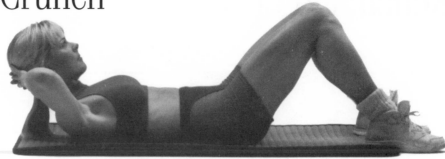

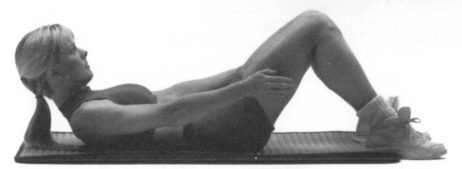

SET-UP:

Lie on your back with your knees bent, feet flat on the floor, hip-width apart and a comfortable distance from your buns. Place your hands behind your head, fingertips touching but not laced together, thumbs behind your ears. Round your elbows outward, tuck your chin a small ways toward your chest, and pull your abs inward.

MOVE:

Count 1: Do a Basic Crunch by curling your head, neck, and chest up and forward off the floor and hold for a moment. *Count 2*: Extend your arms out along the sides of your thighs and hold for a moment. *Count 3*: Curl your body a small way farther upward toward your knees and hold a moment. *Count 4*: Place your hands back behind your head and return to the starting position.

MIND BODY CONNECTION:

Performed correctly, this move is made up of four separate, distinct movements and should take four slow counts to complete. You will feel the strongest pull through your abs when you lift upward for the second time.

VARIATIONS:

- To make this exercise easier, omit the second lift upward (Count 3).
- To make this exercise harder, hold each phase for a slow count of two so the exercise takes a total of eight slow counts to complete.

FORM TIPS:

- Don't pull on your head and neck, especially as you lift up higher for Count 3 of the movement.
- Keep all movements slow and distinct; never bounce or jerk from one phase to the next.

Reach and Crunch

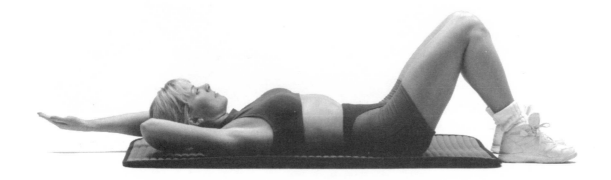

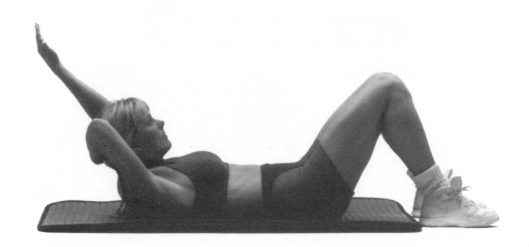

SET-UP:

Lie on your back with your knees bent, feet hip-width apart, flat on the floor, and a comfortable distance from your buns. Place your right hand behind your head, thumb behind your ear, and hold your elbow outward. Extend your left arm straight back behind you so that your upper arm is alongside your ear. Tuck your chin a small way toward your chest and pull your abs inward.

MOVE:

Curl your head, neck, and shoulder blades up off the floor. Hold for a moment at the top of the movement then lower slowly to the start. Switch arms and do an equal number of repetitions.

MIND BODY CONNECTION:

Pretend you are holding an exercise band in your outstretched hand that's attached to the floor. As you pull upward, imagine it adds resistance to the exercise.

VARIATIONS:

• To make this more challenging, extend both arms overhead.
• To make this less challenging, extend your arm straight up over your chest.

FORM TIPS:

• In order to avoid neck strain, make sure your neck remains relaxed and aligned.
• Don't help yourself by swinging your outstretched arm.

Double Crunch

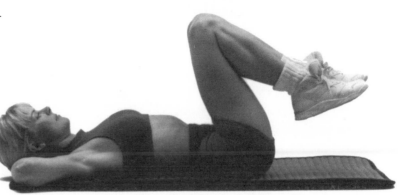

SET-UP:

Lie on your back with your hands behind your head, fingertips touching, thumbs behind your ears. Bend your knees and lift your legs so that your knees are directly over your hips and your lower legs are parallel to the floor. Pull your abs inward and press your back into the floor.

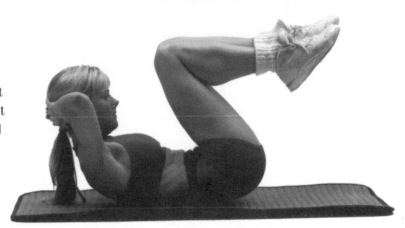

MOVE:

Curl your head, neck, and shoulders up off the floor as you simultaneously lift your hips slightly off the floor so that your knees move a few inches in toward your middle. Hold a moment at the top of the movement and slowly lower to the start.

MIND BODY CONNECTION:

Imagine your *rectus abdominis* is a sheet and you are trying to fold it so that the four corners meet in the middle.

VARIATIONS:

For more of a challenge:

- Hold the up position for a slow five count.
- Pulse 5 to 10 times in the up position by moving your upper and lower body a small distance up and down.
- To make this exercise easier, keep your lower body stationary as you move your upper body.

FOCUS ON FORM:

Don't pull on your neck by drawing your elbows inward to touch your knees! Keep your elbows held outward and your knees directly over your hips.

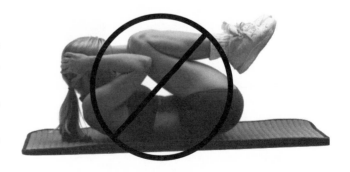

FORM TIPS:

- The object of this exercise is not to touch your elbows to your knees, so avoid drawing your elbows inward or pulling on your neck.
- Keep your knees directly aligned over your hips throughout this exercise.
- Avoid overarching your lower back as you return to the start.

Reverse Crunch

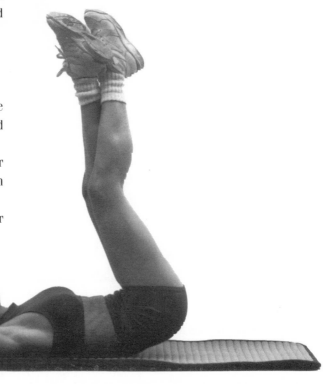

SET-UP:
Lie on your back with your legs up off the floor directly over your hips and your legs extended straight upward. Cross your ankles and bend your knees slightly. Place your hands behind your head, thumbs behind your ears, and extend your elbows outward. Relax your neck and shoulders, and pull your abs inward.

MOVE:
Lift your tailbone 1 or 2 inches straight off the floor so that your feet move directly upward toward the ceiling. Hold a moment and lower slowly.

MIND BODY CONNECTION:
Pretend you're trying to touch the ceiling with your feet. This is a very small, slow, careful move. Done correctly, there is a minimum of leg movement and your hips shouldn't rock backward at all.

VARIATIONS:
If you find this move too difficult:
- Grasp the back edges of an exercise mat or stable object such as the underside of a couch or stuffed chair.
- Try lifting just one leg at a time; bend your other knee so that your foot is flat on the floor. Do an equal number of reps with each leg.
- To make this exercise harder, and to bring your waist into play, try this "obliques" version: with your knees bent and legs off the floor, widen your legs as far to the sides as your flexibility will allow. Perform a reverse crunch while holding your legs in this position.

FORM TIPS:
- Keep your shoulders relaxed and down; don't involve your upper body at all.
- This move is small and precise; you don't have to lift very high to feel this exercise!

Chapter 6

Your Waist

The word "waist" was coined by the fashion industry to standardize middle-body measurements. Contrived though it may be, it's a useful term to describe the point where your stomach tapers inward.

For perfect middle muscles, a trim, clearly defined waistline is a must—a natural connection between sculpted abs and firmly toned lower-back muscles. A contoured waistline also creates symmetry between your upper and lower body, thereby balancing your proportions. There's nothing like a whittled waist to make your shoulders appear broader and your hips and buns more shapely—that hourglass figure.

Working your waistline muscles with the exercises in this chapter helps eliminate the spare tire around your middle by firming and sculpting them. Keep in mind that besides out-of-condition muscles, excess body fat also contributes to that spare tire. Fat burning aerobic workouts combined with a healthy, sensible diet will help decrease body fat and uncover a beautifully toned waistline.

Whenever you rotate or bend at the spine, you use your obliques, the main muscles that cross through and shape your waist area. The best way to work these muscles is by doing exercises that involve twisting or bending to the side. The exercises in this chapter do just that. By including at least one of them in every *Abs of Steel* routine you do, you will help deflate that spare tire and trim inches from your waist.

A Word About Form

All of the exercises in this chapter involve twisting and side-bending movements of the spine, movements designed to zero in on your oblique muscles. Doing these exercises correctly may take some practice, but as your muscles grow stronger you will have an easier time with correct technique. Here are some tips that may help:

- Your arm positioning should remain constant relative to your shoulders for all of these exercises. For instance, always keep your elbows wide—rather than drawing your elbows inward—when doing rotational crunch-style exercises.
- Your neck should remain relaxed, elongated, and in line with rest of your spine.
- Lead any twisting or side-bending movements with your shoulder rather than your elbow so that you are working from the waist and abs rather than simply moving your arms from side-to-side.
- Always exhale through your mouth when you are exerting an effort and inhale through your nose when you're releasing the effort. For most exercises that means exhaling as you lift upward and inhaling as you lower to the start.

If you feel a strong pull, or contraction, on both sides of your waist, you are doing an exercise correctly. Don't worry, we'll give you form tips in the description of each exercise.

How To Use These Exercises

Most of the exercises in this chapter include some flexion, or forward bending, of your spine. Because your *rectus abdominis* is the main mover of forward flexion, it's important to "pre-exhaust" this muscle with crunches in order to better isolate your obliques with rotational crunching and side-bending exercises.

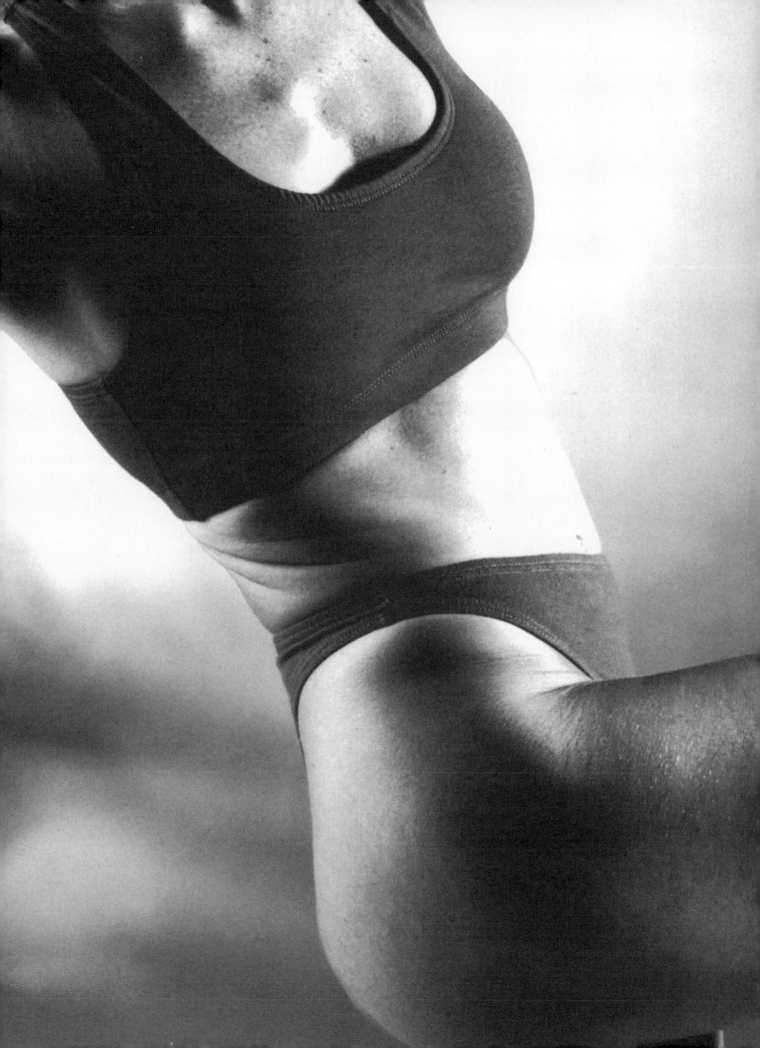

Doing the exercises in the previous chapter before you do the exercises in this chapter allows you to better isolate your obliques and work them to their fullest.

The number of sets and repetitions you will do varies depending on your skill and fitness level, but, in general, you will include 1 to 3 sets of 12 to 20 repetitions, 2 to 3 times a week, of "oblique muscle" training in any **Abs of Steel** routine you do. Most **Abs of Steel** routines allow 30 to 90 seconds rest between each set; long enough to allow your muscles to recover, but not so long that you lose the intensity of your workout. The *Routines* chapter (p. 76) will help you determine the precise number of reps, sets, and exercises you should do for maximum results. Assuming you don't have a great deal of body fat covering your waist, you should notice drastic improvements in about four weeks. Even if you do have a bit of excess body fat, these exercises will still noticeably improve the appearance of your waistline.

Anatomy

Your *internal* and *external obliques* are the topmost of all of your abdominal muscles. In addition to aiding your *rectus abdominis* in flexing, or forward bending of the spine, they are also responsible for any twisting and side-bending movements of your torso. Because the fibers of your oblique muscles are interwoven and wrap all the way around your torso, they provide a lot of lower-back support.

The *external obliques* originate at the side of your lower ribs, run diagonally across your torso, and attach on the fibrous edges of your *rectus abdominis*

muscle. The left *external oblique* is activated when you twist or bend to the right; the right *external oblique* is activated when you twist or bend to the left.

The *internal obliques* run at right angles to, and underneath, the *external obliques.* They are called upon whenever you twist or bend to the same side. In other words, when you twist to the right, your right *internal oblique* contracts, and vice versa.

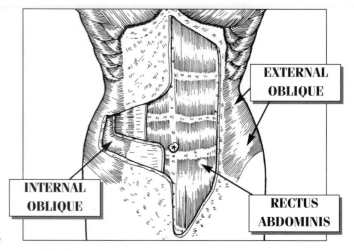

The Exercises in This Chapter

1. Rotational Crunch
2. Double Rotation
3. Sustained Rotation
4. Slow Bicycle
5. Iron Cross
6. Side Crunches
7. Side Sweeps
8. Twisters

Rotational Crunch

SET-UP:

Lie on your back with your knees bent, feet hip-width apart, flat on the floor, and a comfortable distance from your buns. Place your hands behind your head so that your thumbs are behind your ears. *Don't lace your fingers together.* Hold your elbows out wide and slightly tuck your chin toward your chest. Gently pull your abdominals in toward your spine and tilt your pelvis upward.

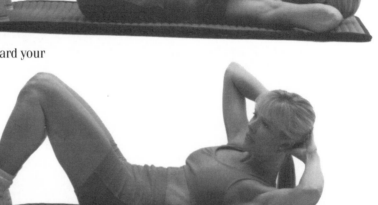

MOVE:

Curl your head, neck, and shoulder blades up off the floor. As you curl upward, move your right shoulder toward your left knee by twisting from your middle. (You don't have to touch your elbow to your knee, so don't draw your elbow inward.) Hold a moment and lower to the start. For the next rep, move your left shoulder toward your right knee, again twisting from the middle. Continue alternating sides until you have completed all reps.

MIND BODY CONNECTION:

As you curl upward and sideways, pretend you are trying to bump something out of the way with your shoulder.

VARIATIONS:

• To make this exercise more advanced, lift your bent knees off the floor, and cross one ankle over the other.
• You can add more "resistance" to this exercise by reaching with your arm extended rather than using your elbow.

FORM TIPS:

• The movement is done by rotating from your middle, not by pulling your elbow in and across your body. Your elbows should not change position during this exercise, and you should barely be able to see the tips of your elbows out of the corners of your eyes.

FOCUS ON FORM:

Don't pull your elbows inward! This may cause neck strain, and besides, it's not as effective as twisting from your waist by using your middle muscles, particularly the obliques.

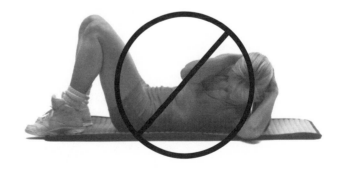

Double Rotation

SET-UP:
Lie on your back with your knees bent, feet hip-width apart, flat on the floor, and a comfortable distance from your buns. Place your hands behind your head, fingertips touching but not laced together, thumbs behind your ears. Hold your elbows outward. Pull your abs inward toward your spine.

MOVE:
Curl your head, neck, and shoulder blades up off the floor. As you curl upward, move your right shoulder toward your left knee by twisting from your middle. Without lowering to the start, rotate to the center and hold a moment before moving your left shoulder toward your right knee. Lower to the start. Start the next repetition by leading up with your left shoulder to right knee.

MIND BODY CONNECTION:
This is one smooth, fluid movement left to right. As you do each repetition, think to yourself, "Twist, center, twist, lower."

VARIATIONS:
• For more of a challenge, add a crunch upward after your twist left and right. (Think, "Twist, center, twist, center and up, lower.")

FORM TIPS:
• Don't pull on your neck by pulling in with your elbows.
• Your movements should be smooth rather than quick and jerky.

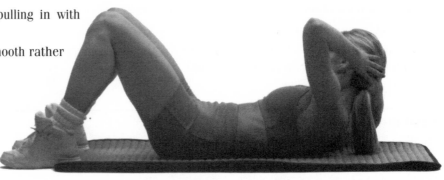

Sustained Rotation

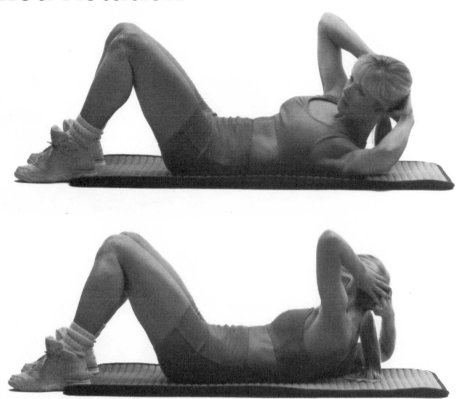

SET-UP:
Lie on your back with your knees bent, feet hip-width apart, flat on the floor, and a comfortable distance from your buns. Place your hands behind your head so that your fingertips are touching and your thumbs are behind your ears. Pull your abs inward. Curl your head, neck, and shoulder blades up off the floor.

MOVE:
From the up position, continuously twist to the left, through the middle and to the right, until you have completed a total of eight left-right rotations. Return to the center and then lower to the start. When you twist to the left, your right elbow will move toward your left side, and when you twist right, your left elbow will move to your right side.

MIND BODY CONNECTION:
Think of your middle spine as a pivot point around which the rest of your body must rotate. As it moves continuously from side to side, everything else remains stationary.

VARIATIONS:
- To make this exercise harder, double the number of rotations to sixteen (eight to each side).
- To make this exercise easier, decrease the number of rotations to four (two to each side).

FORM TIPS:
- Again, your elbows should remain outward throughout the exercise.
- You'll increase the effectiveness of this exercise if you really concentrate on pulling your abs inward as you rotate.

Slow Bicycle

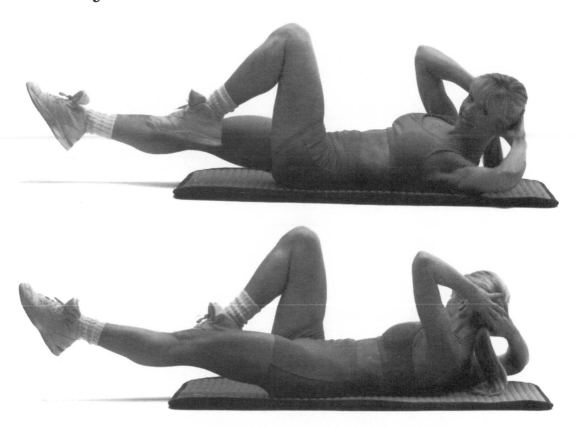

SET-UP:
Lie on your back with your left knee pulled in toward your chest, your right leg fully extended and a few inches off the floor; gently point the toes of both feet. Place your hands behind your head, fingertips touching, and curl your head, neck, and shoulders up off the floor. Rotate from the waist so that your right elbow is near, but not touching, your left knee.

MOVE:
Hold the set-up position for a slow three count, and then switch sides by bending your right knee in toward your chest and extending your left leg out as you rotate your left elbow toward your right knee. Hold for a slow three count before rotating back to the start. Complete all reps before lowering to the floor.

MIND BODY CONNECTION:
Think of pedaling a bike up a very steep hill with your legs.

VARIATIONS:
For more of a challenge:
• Move slowly though the rotation so it, too, takes three slow counts to complete.
• Hold each position for a slow count of five.
For less of a challenge:
• Hold each position for two slow counts.
• Don't extend your leg all the way out.

FORM TIPS:
• All movements should be slow, smooth, and deliberate.
• Hold your extended leg up off the floor only a few inches and keep it directly in line with your hip.

Iron Cross

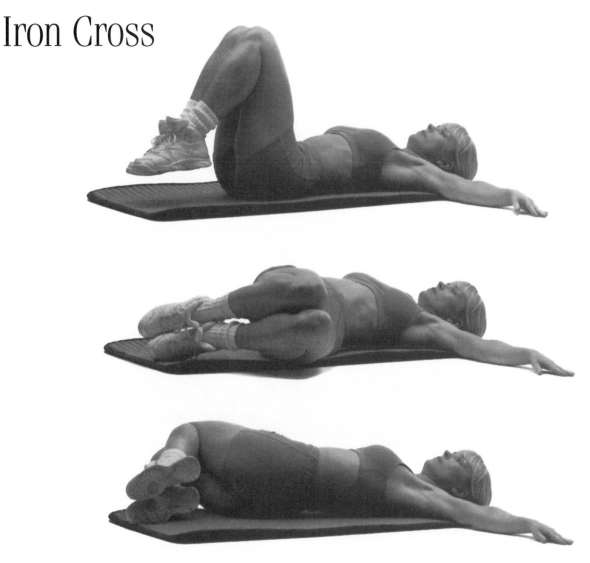

SET-UP:
Lie on your back with your knees bent, legs together and feet a few inches off the floor so that your thighs are perpendicular to the floor and positioned directly over your hips. Extend your arms straight out to the side at shoulder level. Pull your abs inward and press your lower back firmly into the floor.

MOVE:
Pull your abs even further inward and, leading with your knees, slowly lower your bent legs toward the floor to your left side. Depending on your flexibility, they may or may not reach the floor. Lift them back up to the start by pulling your abs inward. Repeat to the right.

MIND BODY CONNECTION:
Think of doing the can-can dance very slowly. Control the movement with your abdominal and oblique muscles rather than your legs or mere momentum.

VARIATIONS:
- For a real challenge, straighten your legs up over your hips and lower them from side to side. Only attempt this variation if your lower back is strong and flexible enough to do so.
- To make this exercise easier, start with your feet flat on the floor.

FORM TIPS:
- Keep your neck and shoulders relaxed.
- Do this move slowly so that your abs, rather than your legs, do the majority of the work.

Side Crunches

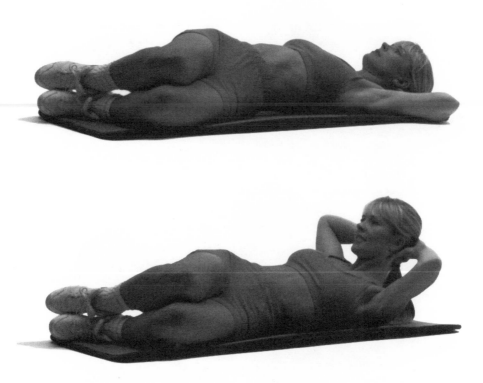

SET-UP:
Lie on your back with your knees bent and your feet and legs together. Anchor both shoulders and your entire upper back firmly to the floor. Roll your hips to the left and lower your legs to the floor on your left side. Place your hands behind your head, fingertips touching but not laced together, thumbs behind your ears. Pull your abs inward.

MOVE:
Curl your head, neck, and shoulders off the floor. Hold a moment before returning to the start. Once you have completed all reps, roll your hips to the right and do an equal number of reps.

MIND BODY CONNECTION:
Pretend there is someone gently pressing down on your thighs to hold them securely in place.

VARIATIONS:
- To make this move more difficult, pulse 5 to 10 times in the up position.
- To make this move easier, only lower your legs about halfway to the floor.

FORM TIPS:
- You may not be able to lift up as high as you can when doing other crunching-type movements. Don't force it. Curl only as high as your flexibility will comfortably allow.

Side Sweeps

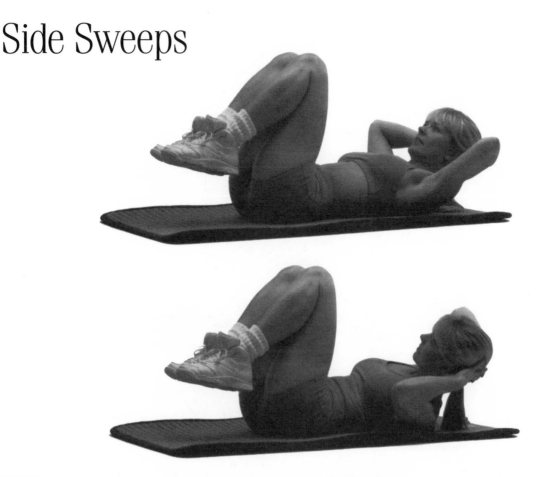

SET-UP:
Lie on your back with your knees bent, feet up off the floor so that your knees are directly over your hips, and your lower legs are relaxed. Gently point your toes. Place your hands behind your head with your thumbs behind your ears and your elbows rounded outward. Curl your head, neck, and shoulder blades up off the floor.

MOVE:
Bend at your waist to the left so that your left elbow moves toward your left hip. Hold a moment and move through the starting position so that your right elbow moves toward your right hip. Continue alternating sides. Complete all reps before lowering to the floor.

MIND BODY CONNECTION:
Think of lengthening the side of your waist opposite to the one you are bending toward.

VARIATIONS:
- Pulling your left hip toward your left elbow places even more emphasis on your obliques.
- For even more of a challenge, do a Basic Crunch to the center between each Side Sweep.
- If you find this exercise too difficult, lower to the floor between each Side Sweep.

FORM TIPS:
- Move your elbow to the side by bending from your waist rather than tilting your neck from side to side.

Twisters

SET-UP:
Sit up very tall with your legs straight out in front of you and hip-width apart, toes relaxed. Extend your arms out to the side at shoulder level. Pull all of your middle muscles in toward your spine.

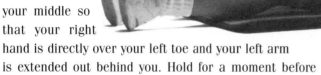

MOVE:
Pull your middle muscles in even more and twist from your middle so that your right hand is directly over your left toe and your left arm is extended out behind you. Hold for a moment before twisting to the left.

MIND BODY CONNECTION:
Imagine your spine is an immovable steel rod anchored to the floor that your body must pivot around. When you twist, you should be able to see the wall to your side. This is also an excellent move for improving posture and spinal flexibility.

VARIATIONS:
- If you need more of a challenge, try this version: once you have twisted to the side, round your middle by pulling your abs inward and reaching forward, trying to touch your left toe if your flexibility allows (your flexibility may prevent you from actually touching your toe, but reach as close to it as you comfortably can). Hold a moment before lifting up tall and twisting to the opposite side.
- If you find this move too difficult, bend your knees about six inches or stop briefly in the center between "twists."

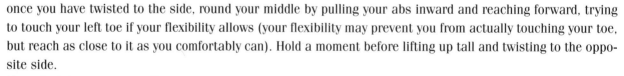

FORM TIPS:
- Concentrate on keeping your buns anchored to the floor, especially as you twist from one side to the other.
- Keep your head and neck in line with the rest of your body as you move.

Chapter 7

Stretching Out

With all this talk about firming and shaping your muscles, it's time to think about stretching them as well. Flexibility training is the ideal complement to target toning. Whereas the exercises in the previous chapters sculpt and shape your middle muscles, the exercises in this chapter will lengthen and loosen them.

Many middle-muscle exercises are considered, quite literally, a pain in the neck. By the time you complete your workout, your neck can often feel tired and achy. Of course, if you are exercising correctly, neck strain should be minimal. However, some amount of stiffness is normal, especially if you are new to **Abs of Steel** training. By performing a good neck stretch at the end of your training session, you will reduce muscle soreness and help prevent injuries from occurring. That way, it's your middle muscles that feel worked—not your neck. The same goes for your shoulders, back, hips, thighs, or any other part of your body that you use even minimally when doing abdominal exercises.

When you target tone a muscle, it responds to the demands placed on it by contracting. You feel this contraction in the form of tension or a strong pull through the working muscle. Given enough work on a regular basis, the muscle grows stronger and firmer. The stronger it gets, the more capable it is of handling exercise. That is why, when you first try a middle-muscle, target-toning exercise, it may be difficult to perform, but after a few weeks of training, it's no sweat. Once you've been working out a while, you'll need to challenge yourself with more difficult variations of each exercise, more advanced routines, and special exercise techniques in order to continue reaping maximum benefits.

Stretching performs the exact opposite function of target toning. Working muscles need a time-out. They've done their job, now they deserve a break! Stretching elongates and relaxes muscles, allowing them to regroup and renew in preparation for the next workout. An **Abs of Steel** training session without a stretch is like having a job without vacations, weekends, and holidays!

Stretching out is also a good way to wind down after a hard workout. It gives you a chance to mentally review what you've done and to think about what you want to do the next time you train. Or you can just let go, allowing your mind and body relax. Many experts believe that this meditative quality is the most important aspect of the postworkout stretch.

Stretching Basics

When performing a stretching exercise, never push it to the point of pain. Ease, rather than force yourself, into a position, and only move into a stretch as much as you comfortably can. You may be able to get into a stretching position pretty easily, but if you can't, don't get discouraged. Do the best you can or try the less difficult version of the stretch until you are more limber. You'll find that some muscles are more limber than others.

Don't "bounce" the muscle up and down in the stretched position or use quick, jerky movements. This increases your risk of injury and may actually cause the muscle to shorten and tighten up. Instead, hold each stretch for at least thirty seconds, concentrating on reaching and lengthening as you do so. Gradually increase the amount of time you hold each stretch to sixty seconds.

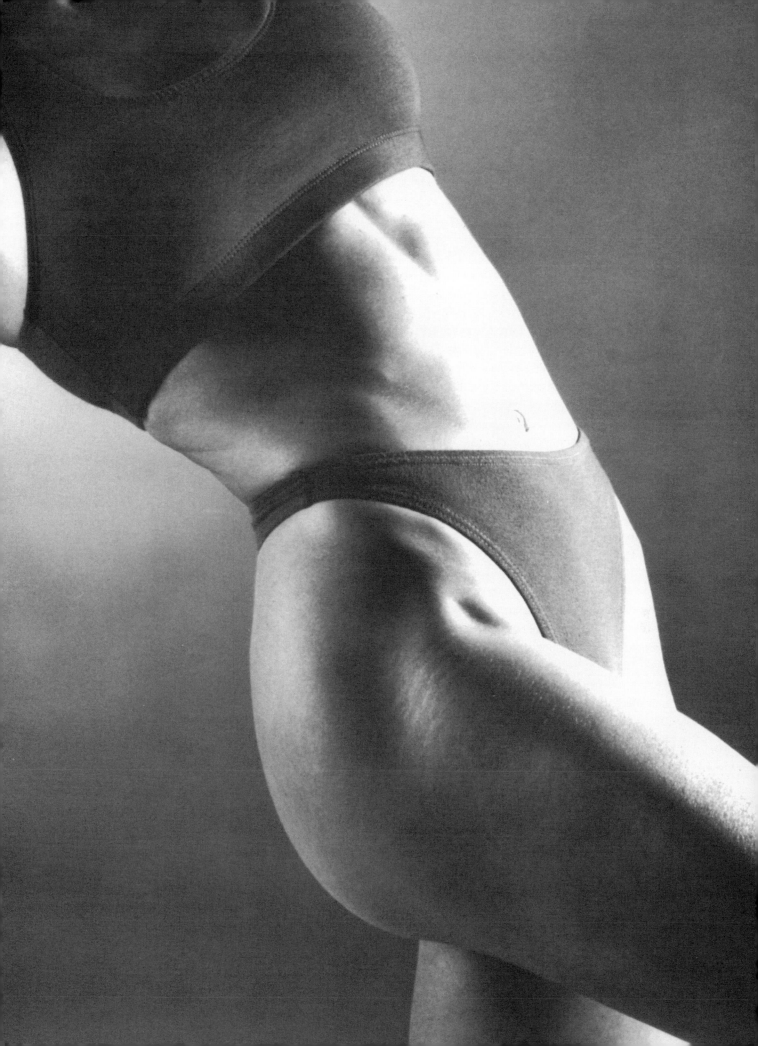

Proper breathing is a very important part of stretching correctly. You'll feel more relaxed and get more out of the stretch. Inhale through your nose for two counts as you move into a stretch and then exhale through your mouth for two counts as you hold it. Keep breathing slowly and deeply as you stay in the stretched position. Never hold your breath! This deprives your muscles of much-needed oxygen and makes it harder to stay loose.

Try to concentrate on the muscle that you are stretching while relaxing the rest of your body. If you're stretching out your lower back, for instance, focus on how those muscles feel. When you breathe, try to imagine air and oxygen quietly streaming into your lower-back muscles. Picture the stretching muscles letting go and giving way: relaxing, lengthening, and loosening. "Listen" for the precise moment your lower back releases all the built-up tension both from your workout and everyday life. Practice this mind/body technique with every stretch you do. After a while, it will become second nature.

You need only do one repetition of each stretch. However, if you feel a particular body part needs special attention or a certain stretch feels especially good, by all means go ahead and do it an extra time or two. Although you can move from one stretch into the next without a break, it's OK to rest for a minute or so between stretches. You might want to do this if you are new to the *Abs of Steel* stretch or your muscles are especially tight.

How To Use These Stretches

Individually, the exercises in this chapter target-stretch an area that you use directly or indirectly in your *Abs of Steel* training. Together, they form a total body stretch, designed to leave you feeling loose and relaxed at the end of each workout. You should do the same routine at the end of every training session regardless of how advanced an exerciser you are. When you get to the *Routines* chapter (p. 76), you'll notice that stretching exercises aren't included in the routine. Nonetheless, you should do at least some of the recommended stretches at the end of every workout. If you do them in the order they're described, one stretch flows right into the next. Once you are familiar with the routine, it shouldn't take you more than six minutes to complete.

You won't have to constantly change the stretches you do the way you change your middle-muscle, target-toning exercises. That's because as your flexibility improves, you develop a greater ability to hold a stretch and elongate your muscles.

Never stretch a "cold" muscle. Always do your *Abs of Steel* stretches after you've completed your middle-muscle workout, or after an aerobic workout. Stretching is more effective when your body temperature is slightly elevated and there's increased blood flow into your working muscles. Your muscles also become more pliable and "receptive" to stretching after they've been moving a while.

The Exercises In This Chapter

1. The Pretzel
2. Hamstring Stretch
3. Knee Crossover
4. The Child
5. Reach Through
6. Side Stretch
7. Ear To Shoulder
8. Thigh Stretch

The Pretzel

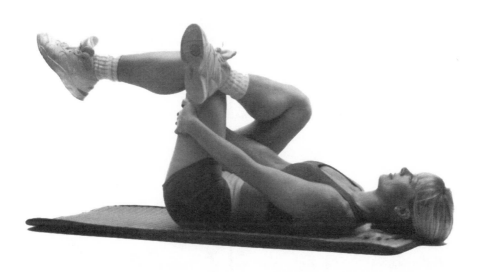

STRETCHES:
Buns, lower back, outer thigh.

SET-UP & MOVE:
Lie on your back and bend your knees. Lift your legs so that your knees are directly over your hips and your lower legs are parallel to the floor. Cross your right ankle over the top of your left thigh. Clasp both hands around the back of your left thigh and pull back with a gentle, steady pressure. As you hold this position, you'll feel the stretch spread through your left bun and outer hip and through the center of your lower back. Repeat to the other side.

VARIATIONS:
- If this is too much of a stretch for you, just position your legs without pulling backward with your hands.
- If you wish to increase the stretch, loop a towel around your left thigh and grasp an end in each hand. Pull back on the towel with a steady, even pressure.

FORM TIPS:
- Don't lift your head off the floor; keep your shoulders relaxed and down.
- Don't arch your lower back off the floor.

Hamstring Stretch

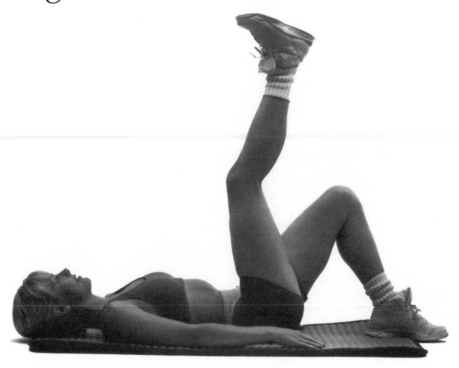

STRETCHES:
Back of your thigh.

SET-UP & MOVE:
Lie on your back with your left knee bent, foot flat on the
floor and a comfortable distance from your buns. Bending
your knee slightly, extend your right leg straight out in
front of you on the floor. Pull your abs inward and press
your back firmly into the floor. Place your arms wherever
they are most comfortable. Slowly raise your right leg off
the floor as high as you can without allowing your back or
buns to lift off the floor. As you hold this position, you'll
feel a stretch through the length of the back of your thigh.
Lower slowly and repeat with your left leg.

VARIATIONS:
• For more of a stretch, clasp your hands around
  the back of your thigh and pull backward with a
  steady, gentle pressure.
• For less of a stretch, bend your knee slightly.

FORM TIPS:
• If you feel any discomfort in your lower back, back
  off the stretch a bit or bend your knee even more.

Knee Crossover

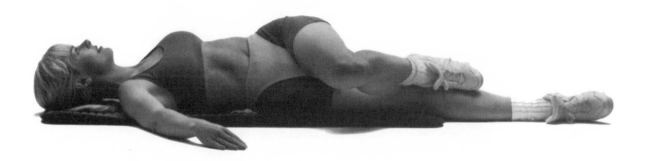

STRETCHES:
Lower and upper back; hips, buns, outer thigh.

SET-UP & MOVE:
Lie on your back with your left knee bent, foot flat on the floor and a comfortable distance from your buns. Extend your right leg straight out along the floor. Place your hands wherever they're comfortable. Keeping your back and shoulders firmly anchored to the floor, roll your left hip off the floor and move your left knee across your body, pressing it to the right and downward. If possible, it should touch the floor on the right side. As you hold this position, the stretch will spread up into your shoulder and down into your lower back, hips, and buns. Pull your abs inward to return to the center; repeat to the other side.

VARIATIONS:
• To intensify the stretch, you can place your right hand on the outside of your knee and gently apply downward pressure.

• To ease up on the stretch, bend both knees and drop them both to one side, then the other.

FORM TIPS:
• Don't force the stretch.
• If you feel any lower-back discomfort, do the less intense version of this move.

The Child

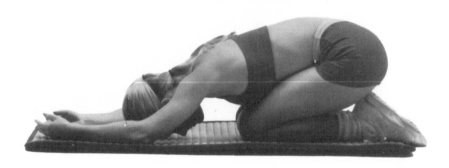

STRETCHES:
Entire length of spine, especially the lower back.

SET-UP & MOVE:
Kneel on your hands and knees with your entire spine aligned. Sit back on your heels or as far back as you comfortably can, stretching through your extended arms and shoulders. As you hold this position, you'll feel a mild stretch along the length of your spine.

VARIATIONS:
- To stretch even more of your spine, lean slightly to the right for a lateral stretch. Hold. Repeat to the left.
- If you find this stretch too difficult, try the following stretch. It has a similar, though milder, effect: lie on your back and gently hug your knees to your chest.

FORM TIPS:
- Pulling your abs up into your spine will increase the effectiveness of this move.
- Breathe deeply and relax!

Reach Through

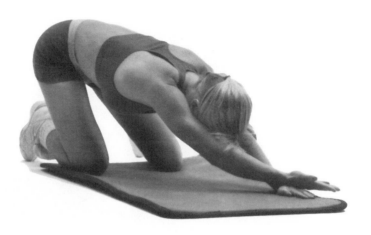

STRETCHES:
Your obliques, shoulder, arm, and lower back.

SET-UP & MOVE:
Kneel with your knees hip-width apart and place your right hand, palm up, on top of your left hand. Look down at the floor so that the back of your neck is lengthened and is in line with the rest of your spine; pull your abs inward. Lift your right hand up about an inch and reach toward the opposite wall as you lean your weight into your right hip. Repeat to the left.

FORM TIPS:
- Lean your weight into your opposite hip rather than sitting back onto your heels.
- Holding your abs inward increases the stretch.

Side Stretch

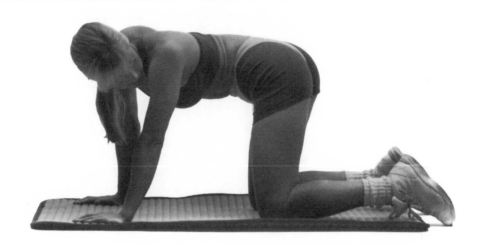

STRETCHES:
Your obliques, lower back.

SET-UP & MOVE:
Kneel on your hands and knees with your knees hip-width apart and your arms shoulder-width apart, weight balanced evenly on your palms and feet. Look down at the floor so that the back of your neck is lengthened and in line with the rest of your spine; pull your abs inward. Look over your left shoulder and cock your left hip forward. Bend your waist to the left and look behind you until you can just see your left foot. As you hold this stretch, you will feel the opposite side, from your shoulder to your hip, lengthen and stretch. Slowly return to center before repeating to the right.

FORM TIPS:
- If you concentrate on keeping your abdominals pulled inward, this will increase the effectiveness of this move.
- Keep your weight balanced evenly on all fours.
- Don't hunch your shoulders.

Ear to Shoulder

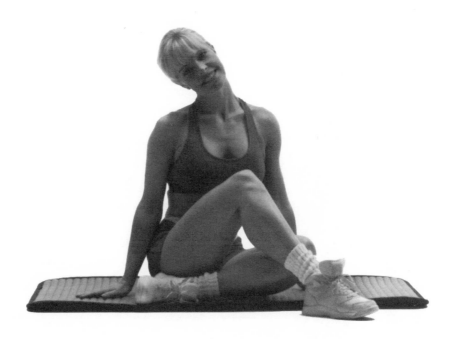

STRETCHES:
Your neck muscles and the top of your shoulders.

SET-UP & MOVE:
Sit up tall in a comfortable, relaxed position. Gently press your shoulders downward and backward. Slowly tip your right ear down toward your right shoulder. As you hold this position, you'll feel the stretch travel down the length of your neck to the top of your shoulder. Repeat to the other side.

VARIATIONS:
- To increase the intensity of the stretch, place your right hand on your head just over your left ear and gently assist your head downward.
- To lessen the intensity of this move, look to the side, as if you are shaking your head "no" in an exaggerated manner and hold.

FORM TIPS:
- Avoid hunching your shoulders.
- Don't allow your chin to drop forward toward your chest.

Thigh Stretch

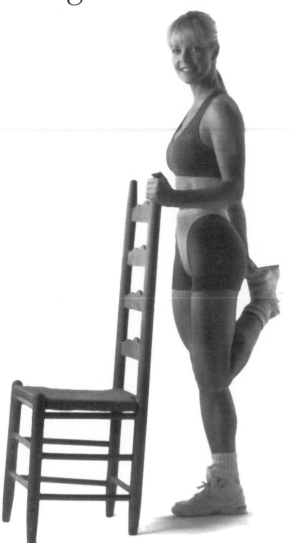

VARIATIONS:
- Holding higher up on the foot, near your ankle, increases the stretch.
- An easier version of this stretch: lie on your side, bring your left heel to your buns and grasp your ankle with your left hand.

FORM TIPS:
- Don't lean forward to increase the stretch; instead, stand up taller and tuck your pelvis slightly forward by gently squeezing your buttocks.
- Avoid arching your lower back.

FOCUS ON FORM:
Don't arch your lower back or lean forward. Instead, stand up tall and gently squeeze your buns together to increase the stretch.

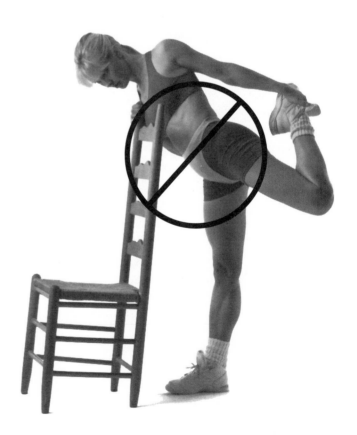

STRETCHES:
The front of your thigh and your hip flexors.

SET-UP & MOVE:
Stand up tall and, if you need to, hold onto a chair or some other sturdy object with your left hand for support. Flex your left foot and bend your left knee back behind you so that your heel moves toward your buns. Grasp the top of your left foot with your right hand and gently press your heel even further into your buns. As you hold this stretch, it will gradually spread upward to the top of your thigh and downward to the top of your knee. Repeat with your right leg.

Chapter 8

The Abs of Steel Routines

Now that you have reviewed the **Abs of Steel** moves, let's put them all together. The routine you do is just as vital to your success as the exercises themselves. For optimal results, it's crucial to do the right amount of exercises in correct order. That is where the **Abs of Steel** routines come in.

As we've told you, the **Abs of Steel** system takes a three-dimensional approach to middle-muscle training. For complete target toning of your middle, you must include at least some of the exercises from each of the exercise chapters on a regular basis (*Stabilization and Awareness, Your Lower Back, Your Abdominals, Your Waist*). If you neglect one group of exercises entirely, you won't see improvements as quickly.

On the following pages, we have laid out some **Abs of Steel** routines for you. They will help you get started. Once you've tried our routines for a while and you get a sense of what works for you, by all means, feel free to be creative! Invent your own routines by using the exercises, variations, and techniques we've given you.

Common Questions

Before you jump in, take some time to review the following, frequently asked questions about **Abs of Steel** training and abdominal training in general. The answers we've outlined here should clear up any confusion you have about the right way to get your middle muscles into tiptop, rock hard condition.

*How do I know whether I'm a beginner, intermediate, or advanced **Abs of Steel** exerciser?*

To get a read on what kind of shape your middle muscles are in, perform the strength and flexibility tests in Chapter 2, *How to Use This Book* (p. 10). They will provide you with useful information on your current condition. Even if you decide not to take the tests you should consider yourself a beginner if you haven't done much target toning with your middle muscles. If you've been target toning your abs between one and three months, start with the intermediate routines; if you've been exercising them consistently for more than three months, you're probably ready for the advanced routines.

Remember, these are just guidelines. *Listen to your body.* It will tell you when you're working at the proper level.

In what order should I do the exercises?

Exercise sequence is important. Working your middle muscles in a precise order ensures that each muscle group will get the proper amount of work. Do your stabilization and awareness exercises first to warm up your middle muscles and prepare them for the rest of your workout. Do your lower-back exercises next while these muscles are still strong; this also helps warm them up even more thoroughly. Abdominal and waist exercises come next. They complete the strength training portion of your workout.

We haven't included the stretching exercises as part of the **Abs of Steel** routines. You should do at least some of the stretches immediately following every workout, even the shorter routines. Once you learn the entire stretching routine, it doesn't take that long—no more than six minutes. However, if you have limited time, concentrate your efforts on the muscles that are prone to injury or that have a tendency to ache. If your neck bothers you after a middle-muscle workout, for instance, be sure to include the Ear to Shoulder stretch.

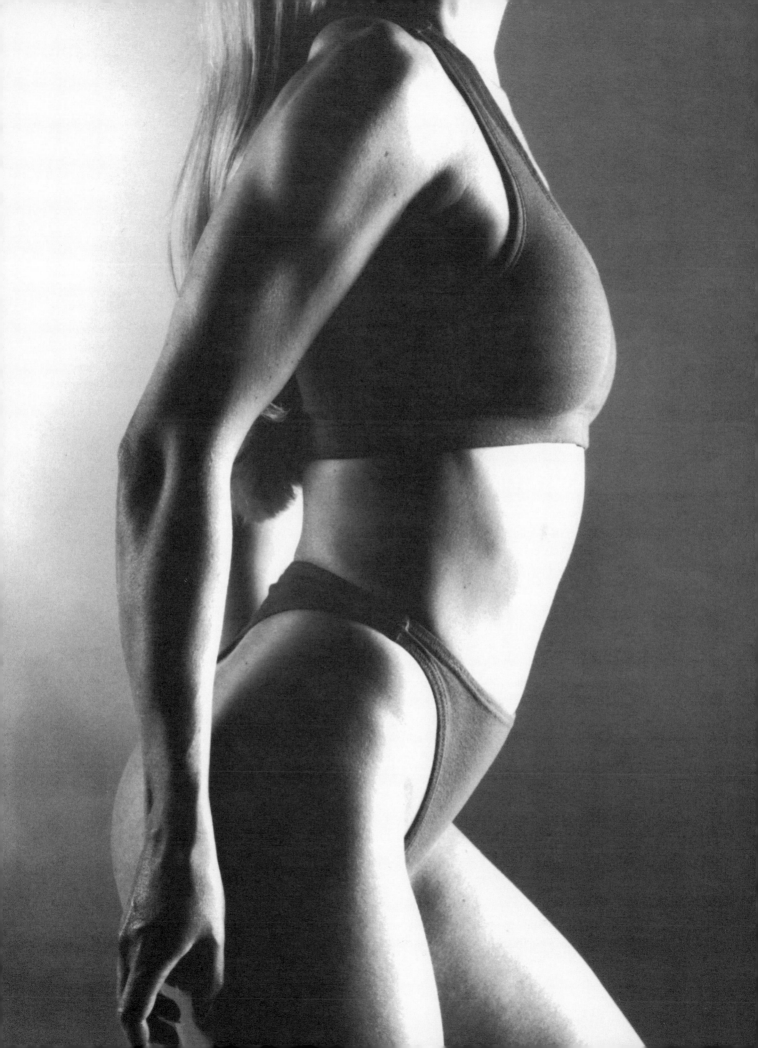

How many reps should I do?

The number of reps necessary for maximum results varies depending on the type and intensity of the exercise. In general, you'll do 5 to 10 reps of stabilization and awareness exercises, 5 to 20 reps of lower-back exercises, and 12 to 20 total repetitions of both abdominal and waist exercises.

In the routines below we suggest a repetition range for each exercise. Start with the least number of suggested reps. When you can complete them with good form, add between one and three repetitions. Once you can do the largest number of recommended reps, and you feel confident you're doing the move correctly, you have several options. You can move into a more difficult variation of the same exercise, increase the number of sets you do per exercise, exchange the exercise for one that has a similar benefit. Or, use one of the special advanced techniques described in the next chapter. When your entire routine is in need of revamping, simply switch to a different routine.

What if you find the minimum suggested number of reps too much for you? Don't get discouraged! Just do what you can, rest as frequently as you need to, and gradually increase your reps until you reach the minimum. You can always try the variations of the exercises that make them easier. Remember, it's not quantity that counts here—it's quality. Better to do two reps correctly than twenty with poor form.

How many sets should I do?

Start with one set of each exercise. Once you can do the maximum number of recommended reps, one way to increase the intensity of your workout is to increase the number of sets you do per workout. Work up to three sets per exercise. We don't recommend going beyond that because it's very time consuming, and ultimately, there is not much additional benefit. Why spend your entire day working your abs when there are so many other ways to get results?

How much weight should I use?

Most people find that the weight of their own body provides enough resistance for middle-muscle exercises, so unless you're a very advanced exerciser, you probably won't ever need a weight, exercise band, or any other special equipment to do these routines. However, adding external "resistance" or additional weight to some of the exercises can be a very effective target-toning technique. The *Special Advanced Techniques* section in the next chapter outlines exactly how to do this. You'll find that adding weight works best with exercises that target your abdominals and waist.

How much should I rest between sets?

Rest between 30 and 90 seconds between each exercise set. This will allow your muscles enough time to recover so they are strong enough to work their hardest but not so long that you lose the intensity and focus of your workout. You will find that as you become stronger, you won't need as much rest between sets. Some special advanced techniques eliminate rest between sets entirely.

How often should I target tone my abs?

For best results, target tone your abs three to six times a week. *Don't think of your rest days as a waste of time!* They are just as important as your workout days. Your middle muscles need time to recover and repair between workouts. Training them every day isn't a good idea. Overtraining will slow your progress and increase your chance of injury. If you prefer to train more often, try the split routines. They allow you to work opposing muscle groups on alternate days.

If I train consistently, how long will it take to see results?

Although everyone's body responds differently to exercise, most people can expect to see noticeable results from their **Abs of Steel** training in about a month. Results may range from clearly defined muscles to a tighter, flatter tummy. If you have an extra layer of body fat covering your middle, aerobic exercise and a low-fat diet will help speed your progress.

You'll probably feel a difference before you see it. After just a couple of workouts, you'll notice your back will feel stronger and looser, and you won't have as much trouble standing or sitting up straight. Your abdominals and waist muscles will be stronger and more supportive. Eventually, this increased strength and flexibility will translate into improvements you can see in the mirror even if you never shed an ounce of fat.

Timed Routines

Some days you have unlimited time to do a leisurely workout and other days you're lucky if you're able to grab a quick lunch. So it follows that the time you can dedicate to *Abs of Steel* training may vary.

What is the least amount of time you can spend on your *Abs of Steel* program and still get results? As little as five minutes a workout. So long as you make each exercise count by using good form and concentrating on each and every rep, you can still reap target-toning benefits by doing as few as four exercises per workout.

If your schedule allows, you will see results faster if you spend a little longer working your middle muscles. That's why we've also given you 10-, 15-, and 20-minute routines. And if you have more time some days than others, mix and match different timed routines for your level.

Once you've carefully reviewed the descriptions of all the exercises, figure out how much time you want to spend target toning your abs (5, 10, 15, or 20 minutes) and then find the appropriate routine for your level.

5-Minute Routines

BEGINNER

Order	Exercise	Variation	Sets	Reps	Page
1	The Zipper	None	1	5-8	25
2	Pelvic Tilt	None	1	10-20	31
3	Basic Crunch	None	1	10-20	44
4	Rotational Crunch	None	1	5-10 each side	55

INTERMEDIATE

Order	Exercise	Variation	Sets	Reps	Page
1	The Slide	None	1	5-8	20
2	Chair Tilt	None	1	10-15	32
3	Crunch and Curl	None	1	10-20	45
4	Double Rotation	None	1	5-15	56

ADVANCED

Order	Exercise	Variation	Sets	Reps	Page
1	Roll-Up	None	1	5-8	24
2	The Ball	None	1	5-15	38
3	Four-Count Crunch	None	1	5-15	48
4	Slow Bicycle	None	1	5-10 each side	58

10-Minute Routines

BEGINNER

Order	Exercise	Variation	Sets	Reps	Page
1	Static Crunch	None	1	5-8	23
2	Cat-Cow	None	1	8-15	34
3	Press-Up	None	1	5-15	35
4	Basic Crunch	None	1	10-20	44
5	Reverse Crunch	None	1	10-20	51
6	Side Sweeps	None	1	5-10 each side	61

INTERMEDIATE

Order	Exercise	Variation	Sets	Reps	Page
1	Stepping	None	1	5-10 each leg	21
2	The Fulcrum	None	1	5-8 each leg	33
3	Swimming	None	1	10-20 each leg	37
4	Single Straight Leg Crunch	None	1	5-10 each leg	46
5	Reverse Crunch	None	1	10-20	51
6	Side Crunches	None	1	5-10 each side	60

ADVANCED

Order	Exercise	Variation	Sets	Reps	Page
1	Extended Contraction	None	1	5-10	19
2	Chair Tilt	None	1	10-20	32
3	Back Sweep	None	1	5-15	36
4	Double Crunch	None	1	10-20	50
5	Reverse Crunch	"Obliques" version	1	10-20	51
6	Sustained Rotation	None	1	10-20	57

15-Minute Routines

BEGINNER

Order	Exercise	Variation	Sets	Reps	Page
1	Extended Contraction	None	1	5-8	19
2	Static Crunch	None	1	5-8	23
3	Pelvic Tilt	None	1	10-20	31
4	Cat-Cow	None	1	8-15	34
5	Basic Crunch	None	1	10-20	44
6	Reverse Crunch	None	1	10-20	51
7	Rotational Crunch	None	1	5-10 each side	55
8	Iron Cross	None	1	5-10 each side	59

INTERMEDIATE

Order	Exercise	Variation	Sets	Reps	Page
1	Stepping	None	1	5-15 each leg	21
2	The Zipper	None	1	5-15	25
3	Chair Tilt	None	1	10-20	32
4	Swimming	None	1	10-20 each leg	37
5	Crunch and Point	None	1	10-20	47
6	Double Crunch	None	1	10-20	50
7	Double Rotation	None	1	5-15	56
8	Side Crunches	None	1	5-10 each side	60

ADVANCED

Order	Exercise	Variation	Sets	Reps	Page
1	Roll-Up	None	1	5-8	24
2	Negative Push-Ups	None	1	3-8	22
3	The Fulcrum	None	1	5-8 each leg	33
4	Back Sweep	Arms all the way back	1	5-15	36
5	Four-Count Crunch	Increase to six counts	1	5-15	48
6	Double Crunch	None	1	10-20	50
7	Sustained Rotation	None	1	10-20	57
8	Twisters	Reach Forward	1	5-15 each side	62

20-Minute Routines

BEGINNER

Order	Exercise	Variation	Sets	Reps	Page
1	Extended Contraction	None	1	5-8	19
2	The Zipper	None	1	5-15	25
3	Pelvic Tilt	None	1	10-20	31
4	The Ball	None	1	5-15	38
5	Basic Crunch	None	2	10-20	44
6	Reverse Crunch	None	2	10-20	51
7	Rotational Crunch	None	2	10-20	55
8	Double Rotation	None	1	5-10 each side	56
9	Twisters	None	1	5-10 each side	62

INTERMEDIATE

Order	Exercise	Variation	Sets	Reps	Page
1	The Slide	None	1	5-8	20
2	Stepping	None	1	5-10 each leg	21
3	Pelvic Circles	None	1	3-8 each direction	26
4	Chair Tilt	None	1	10-20	32
5	Swimming	None	1	10-20 each side	37
6	Single Straight Leg Crunch	None	2	5-10 each leg	46
7	Double Crunch	None	2	10-20	50
8	Double Rotation	None	1	10-20	56
9	Side Sweeps	None	1	10-20 each side	61

ADVANCED

Order	Exercise	Variation	Sets	Reps	Page
1	Roll-Up	None	1	5-8	24
2	Negative Push-Ups	Hold midrange	1	3-8	22
3	Pelvic Circles	Increase range of motion	1	3-6 each direction	26
4	The Fulcrum	Lying on stomach	1	5-8 each side	33
5	Swimming	Lift higher	1	10-20 each side	37
6	Four-Count Crunch	None	2	5-15	48
7	Reach and Crunch	Both arms extended	2	5-15	49
8	Iron Cross	Legs extended	1	5-10 each side	59
9	Side Crunches	Pulse 5 times at top	1	5-10 each side	60

Two Day Split Routines

5 Minute Per Workout Split Routines

Here's an example of how you can use a two day, split routine: On Monday, do Day One and on Tuesday, do Day Two. Rest on Day Three. Repeat the Day One routine on Thursday and Day Two on Friday. If there's a routine you'd particularly like to focus on, you may repeat that workout a third time on Saturday or Sunday.

BEGINNER

Day 1 - Stabilization and Awareness + Lower-Back Focus

Order	Exercise	Variation	Sets	Reps	Page
1	Extended Contraction	None	1	5-10	19
2	The Zipper	None	1	5-10	25
3	Pelvic Tilt	None	1	10-20	31
4	Press-Up	None	1	10-20	35

Day 2 - Abdominals + Waist Focus

Order	Exercise	Variation	Sets	Reps	Page
1	Basic Crunch	None	1	10-20	44
2	Reverse Crunch	None	1	10-20	51
3	Rotational Crunch	None	1	5-10 each side	55
4	Side Sweeps	None	1	5-10 each side	61

INTERMEDIATE

Day 1 - Stabilization and Awareness + Lower-Back Focus

Order	Exercise	Variation	Sets	Reps	Page
1	The Slide	None	1	5-8	20
2	Roll-Up	None	1	5-8	24
3	Chair Tilt	None	1	10-20	32
4	Swimming	None	1	10-20	37

Day 2 - Abdominals + Waist Focus

Order	Exercise	Variation	Sets	Reps	Page
1	Crunch and Curl	None	1	10-20	45
2	Double Crunch	None	1	10-20	50
3	Double Rotation	None	1	5-15	56
4	Side Crunches	None	1	5-10 each side	60

ADVANCED

Day 1 - Stabilization and Awareness + Lower-Back Focus

Order	Exercise	Variation	Sets	Reps	Page
1	Roll-Up	None	1	5-8	24
2	Pelvic Circles	None	1	3-5 each direction	26
3	The Fulcrum	None	1	3-5 each side	33
4	Back Sweep	None	1	5-15	36

Day 2 - Abdominals + Waist Focus

Order	Exercise	Variation	Sets	Reps	Page
1	Crunch and Point	None	1	10-20	47
2	Four-Count Crunch	Add 2 counts	1	10-20	48
3	Sustained Rotation	None	1	5-10 each side	57
4	Slow Bicycle	None	1	5-10 each side	58

10 Minute Per Workout Split Routines

Do both of the appropriate routines for your level on consecutive days and then take one day off. Repeat the routines and then take the next two days off. If there's an area you'd particularly like to focus on, you may repeat that workout a third time.

BEGINNER

Day 1 - Stabilization and Awareness + Lower-Back Focus

Order	Exercise	Variation	Sets	Reps	Page
1	Extended Contraction	None	1	5-10	19
2	The Slide	None	1	5-10	20
3	Roll-Up	None	1	5-10	24
4	Pelvic Tilt	None	1	10-20	31
5	Swimming	None	1	10-20 each side	37
6	The Ball	None	1	5-15	38

Day 2 - Abdominals + Waist Focus

Order	Exercise	Variation	Sets	Reps	Page
1	Basic Crunch	None	1	10-20	44
2	Single Straight Leg Crunch	None	1	5-10 each side	46
3	Reverse Crunch	None	1	10-20	51
4	Rotational Crunch	None	1	5-10 each side	55
5	Iron Cross	None	1	5-10 each side	59
6	Twisters	None	1	5-10 each side	62

INTERMEDIATE

Day 1 - Stabilization and Awareness + Lower-Back Focus

Order	Exercise	Variation	Sets	Reps	Page
1	Static Crunch	None	1	5-10	23
2	Negative Push-Ups	None	1	5-10	22
3	Pelvic Circles	None	1	3-5 each direction	26
4	Cat-Cow	None	1	10-20	34
5	Press-Up	Lift an additional inch	1	5-15	35
6	Swimming	None	1	10-20 each side	37

Day 2 - Abdominals + Waist Focus

Order	Exercise	Variation	Sets	Reps	Page
1	Basic Crunch	Pulse 5-10 times at top	1	10-20	44
2	Reach and Crunch	None	1	10-20	49
3	Double Crunch	None	1	10-20	50
4	Double Rotation	None	1	5-10 each side	56
5	Side Crunches	None	1	5-10 each side	60
6	Twisters	Reach forward	1	5-10 each side	62

ADVANCED

Day 1 - Stabilization and Awareness + Lower-Back Focus

Order	Exercise	Variation	Sets	Reps	Page
1	Stepping	None	1	5-15 each leg	21
2	Negative Push-Ups	Hold midrange	1	3-8	22
3	Roll-Up	Don't use hands	1	5-10	24
4	The Fulcrum	Lying on floor	1	5-10 each side	33
5	Press-Up	Lift an additional inch	1	5-15	35
6	Back Sweep	Increase range of motion	1	5-15	36

Day 2 - Abdominals + Waist Focus

Order	Exercise	Variation	Sets	Reps	Page
1	Four-Count Crunch	Add 2 counts	1	5-15	48
2	Crunch and Point	Arms at sides	1	10-20	47
3	Reverse Crunch	Obliques version	1	10-20	51
4	Slow Bicycle	None	1	5-10 each side	58
5	Iron Cross	Legs extended	1	5-10 each side	59
6	Twisters	Reach forward	1	5-10 each side	62

Three Day Split Routines

The following beginner, intermediate, and advanced routines are just an example of how you can split up your **Abs of Steel** workout to emphasize one particular muscle group without neglecting the others. Three day splits require six days of training per week. Do not skip that all-important rest day.

Do all three of the appropriate routines for your level in order and then take one day off. Repeat all three routines to complete your **Abs of Steel** training for the week.

BEGINNER

Day 1 - Stabilization and Awareness + Abdominals Focus

Order	Exercise	Variation	Sets	Reps	Page
1	The Slide	None	1	5-8	20
2	The Zipper	None	1	5-8	25
3	Basic Crunch	None	1	10-20	44
4	Reverse Crunch	None	1	10-20	51

Day 2 - Lower Back + Waist Focus

Order	Exercise	Variation	Sets	Reps	Page
1	The Fulcrum	None	1	3-5 each side	33
2	Press-Up	None	1	5-15	35
3	Rotational Crunch	None	1	5-10 each side	55
4	Twisters	None	1	5-10 each side	62

Day 3 - Abdominals + Waist Focus

Order	Exercise	Variation	Sets	Reps	Page
1	Crunch and Point	None	1	10-20	47
2	Double Crunch	None	1	10-20	50
3	Double Rotation	None	1	5-10 each side	56
4	Side Crunches	None	1	5-10 each side	60

INTERMEDIATE

Day 1 - Stabilization and Awareness + Abdominals Focus

Order	Exercise	Variation	Sets	Reps	Page
1	Stepping	None	1	5-15 each leg	21
2	Negative Push-Ups	None	1	3-5	22
3	Reach and Crunch	None	1	10-20	49
4	Reverse Crunch	None	1	10-20	51

Day 2 - Lower Back + Waist Focus

Order	Exercise	Variation	Sets	Reps	Page
1	Pelvic Tilt	None	1	10-20	31
2	Swimming	None	1	10-20 each side	37
3	Slow Bicycle	None	1	5-10 each side	58
4	Side Sweeps	None	1	5-10 each side	61

Day 3 - Abdominals + Waist Focus

Order	Exercise	Variation	Sets	Reps	Page
1	Single Straight Leg Crunch	None	1	10-20	46
2	Double Crunch	None	1	10-20	50
3	Double Rotation	None	1	5-10 each side	56
4	Twisters	Reach forward	1	5-10 each side	62

ADVANCED

Day 1 - Stabilization and Awareness + Abdominals Focus

Order	Exercise	Variation	Sets	Reps	Page
1	Roll-Up	Don't use hands	1	5-8	24
2	Pelvic Circles	None	1	3-5 each direction	26
3	Reach and Crunch	None	1	10-20	49
4	Double Crunch	None	1	10-20	50

Day 2 - Lower Back + Waist Focus

Order	Exercise	Variation	Sets	Reps	Page
1	Chair Tilt	Both feet up	1	10-20	32
2	The Ball	Hold rolled back position	1	10-20 each side	38
3	Slow Bicycle	None	1	5-10 each side	58
4	Iron Cross	Legs straight	1	5-10 each side	59

Day 3 - Abdominals + Waist Focus

Order	Exercise	Variation	Sets	Reps	Page
1	Crunch and Curl	Pulse 5-10 times	1	10-20	45
2	Reverse Crunch	Obliques version	1	10-20	51
3	Side Crunches	Pulse 5-10 times	1	5-10 each side	60
4	Twisters	Reach forward	1	5-10 each side	59

Chapter 9
Breaking Out of Your Routine

Although we've tried to give you a great number and variety of *Abs of Steel* routines in the previous chapter, you may find that none of them suits you. The beauty of our middle-muscle training system is that it can be adapted to suit virtually every exerciser.

On the following pages you will find special routines to address different exercise needs. Even if you don't see your particular problem or condition, that doesn't mean *Abs of Steel* training isn't for you. You should be able to find at least one exercise in every chapter that works for you. Even if you can only do a few reps of a few exercises, stick with it. You will find the results are worth it.

And if you are an advanced exerciser who finds even the more difficult variations of the exercise a breeze we haven't forgotten about you either. The special advanced techniques at the end of this chapter will intensify your workout and give you the results you've been looking for. Here's what to do:

If You're Pregnant ...

Most women can continue to exercise throughout pregnancy with no risk to either themselves or their impending bundle of joy. Many experts claim stronger abdominal muscles make pushing during labor easier and help speed postpartum recovery. However, check with your doctor before beginning this or any other exercise program, particularly if you have a history of diabetes, high blood sugar, high blood pressure, or complicated pregnancy.

After the first trimester (beginning of the fourth month) you should discontinue any exercise where you must lie flat on your back, as this could cause your uterus to compress a major artery. Increased hormones cause your joints and ligaments to relax, so avoid overstretching or any bouncy, jerky movements. Isometric techniques such as holds and pulses should also be dropped from your program because they elevate both your and the baby's blood pressure. Moves that require a great deal of balance should be done with care. Remember, your center of gravity has completely changed.

It's especially important to keep plenty of fluids on hand and to stay comfortably cool. Never exercise to total exhaustion, and stop exercising if any unusual symptoms occur, including pain of any kind, leaking of amniotic fluid, cramping, nausea, faintness, dizziness, heart palpitations, numbness in any part of your body, or decreased fetal activity.

So which *Abs of Steel* exercises are safe and practical to do during pregnancy? You can continue your favorite routines from the *Routines* chapter (p. 76) up until your fourth month, so long as you feel up to it. You may find certain exercises don't feel comfortable; remove them from your routine. Cat-Cow and The Fulcrum (*Your Lower Back* chapter, p. 28) and Twisters (*Your Waist* chapter, p. 52) may be done without modification at any point during your pregnancy, as long as you feel up to it. The Thigh Stretch, The Child, the Reach Through, Side Stretch, and Ear to Shoulder stretches are also safe. Other *Abs of Steel* exercises are ideal for pregnant women when the following modifications are made:

Basic Crunch: Sit with your back propped up by several large pillows. Bend your knees so that your feet are flat on the floor and hip-width apart. Extend your arms in front of you. Curl upward and forward by using your

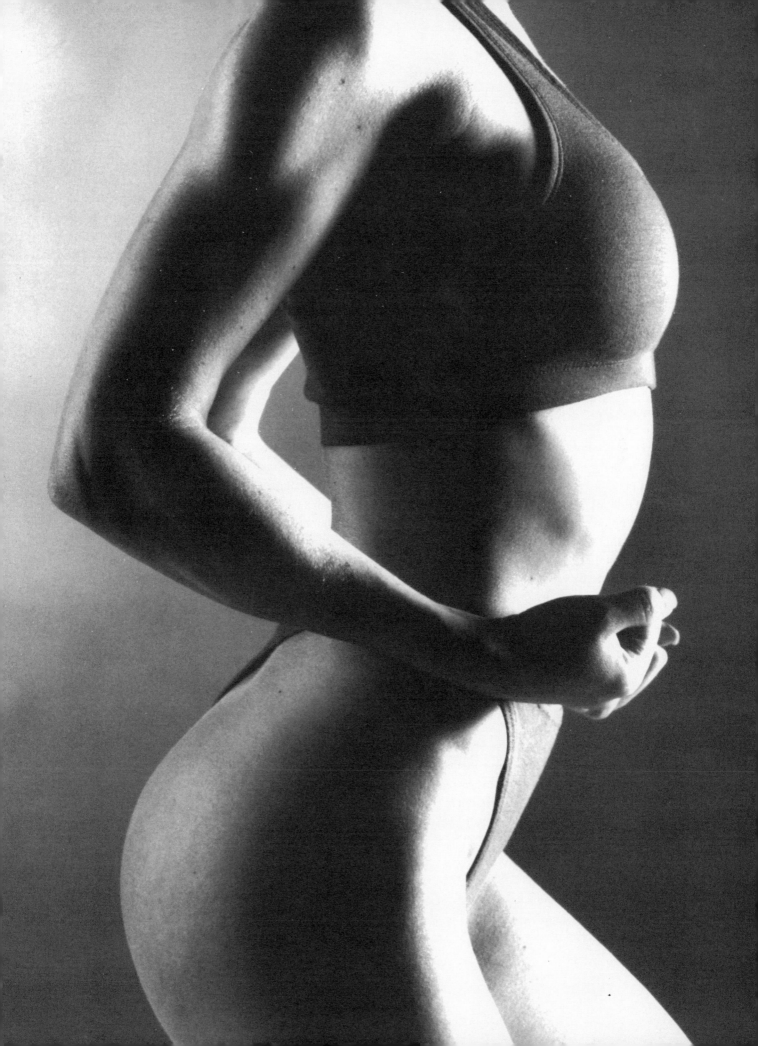

abdominal muscles, always keeping your lower back supported and your head higher than your heart. Slowly return to the start. Do 1 to 3 sets of 10 to 20 reps.

Pelvic Tilt: Lie on your side with your head resting on your outstretched arm. Bend your top knee toward your chest and extend your bottom leg out straight. Do a Pelvic Tilt by gently squeezing your buttocks and tilting your hip bones forward. Return to the start. Do 1 to 3 sets of 10 to 20 reps.

Roll-Up: Stand a few inches away from a wall with your feet hip-width apart, your head and entire back from the top of your shoulders to your tailbone firmly pressed against it. Slowly curl your spine off the wall, one vertebra at a time. Roll down as far as your belly will comfortably allow and then slowly roll back up to the start. Do 1 to 3 sets of 5 to 8 reps.

Side Sweeps: Stand with your feet hip-width apart, your back against a wall. Place your hands behind your head, elbows wide. Bend at your waist to the side as much as you comfortably can by sliding your back along the wall. Sweep through the middle as you side-bend to the other side. Do 1 to 3 sets of 5 to 10 reps each side.

If You Have Chronic Lower-Back Problems ...

If you are currently experiencing lower-back pain, it's a good idea to check with your back-care specialist before beginning any sort of exercise program. Ordinarily, if you are in the throes of a back "episode," it's probably best to wait until the pain subsides before trying to stretch or strengthen the injured muscles.

Any *Abs of Steel* routine you do will help alleviate back pain by strengthening all the muscles which support your spine and by lengthening them and loosening them as well. However, if any one of them leaves your lower-back feeling not quite right—either while you're performing the exercise or afterward—discontinue it and come back to it after you have been training a while. Once your middle muscles are stronger, there's a good chance you'll be able to do all the exercises without pain.

Try the following routine if you have lower-back problems and feel cautious about simply jumping into an *Abs of Steel* workout. This routine was designed to keep your back supported at all times and limit spinal movement. Do this workout 3 to 5 times a week for a month or until your back feels strong enough to move onto a more challenging routine. Or, you can alternate this with another *Abs of Steel* routine.

LOWER-BACK SAFE ROUTINE

Order	Exercise	Variation	Sets	Reps	Page
1	Extended Contraction	None	1	5-8	19
2	The Slide	None	1	5-10	20
3	Pelvic Tilt	None	1	10-20	31
4	The Fulcrum	Lie on your back	1	10-20	33
5	Reverse Crunch	Keep movement small	1	10-20	51
6	Side Sweeps	None	1	5-10 each side	61

Postworkout Stretch: The Pretzel, Hamstring Stretch, Knee Crossover, The Child.

If You're Very Out of Shape ...

For someone who never has worked her middle muscles or who hasn't worked them in a long time, taking the first step can be the hardest, especially if even the beginner routines are too challenging. If you fall into that category, don't get discouraged! You'll see improvements soon enough and feel stronger after just a couple of workouts.

If you can't complete the recommended number of reps in the routines, do what you can, rest, and do some more. You will gradually increase in stamina and strength. Before you know it, you'll be combing through the exercise variations and special advanced techniques! Meanwhile, try the following routine; it was designed for those who need an especially gentle starting point.

FIRST TIMER ROUTINE

Order	Exercise	Variation	Sets	Reps	Page
1	The Zipper	Bend knees	1	2-5	25
2	Static Crunch	None	1	2-5	23
3	Cat-Cow	Upward arch only	1	2-5	34
4	Pelvic Tilt	None	1	3-8	31
5	Basic Crunch	Fold arms across chest	1	3-8	44
6	Iron Cross	Start w/feet flat on floor	1	2-5 each side	59

If You Sit A Lot ...

Anyone who sits at a desk all day knows what it feels like to have an achy back and sore neck. Not to mention what slouching in a chair all day does to your posture.

You can eliminate many of the effects of sitting for long periods of time by making sure your desk area is "ergonomically" correct (ergonomic is just a fancy word for making your work environment work for you).

Your office chair should enable you to sit up straight. It should curve slightly to allow for the slight curve of your lower back. If it doesn't, purchase a lumbar roll at your local pharmacy or medical supply store and place it between the small of your back and the chair; or, you can roll up a thick bath towel for the same effect.

Set your chair height so that when your knees are bent and your feet are flat on the floor, your thighs are parallel to the floor. If your chair won't allow for this, place a book or two under your feet.

If you are working at a computer, situate the screen so that it's at, or slightly above, eye level and about twenty inches away from you. Get a copy holder so you don't strain your neck by constantly hunching over your desk to read.

Here is perhaps the most important tip for those who sit for a living: get up and take frequent breaks. You can modify most of the *Abs of Steel* exercises for a sitting position, including the stretches. Or, if possible, get down on the office floor and do the following "posture-picker-upper" routine (if you get some funny stares from your co-workers, it's OK to wait until you get home before you do it)! Do the variation of each exercise that suits your level.

POSTURE-PICKER-UPPER ROUTINE

Order	Exercise	Variation	Sets	Reps	Page
1	Roll-Up	None	1	3-8	24
2	The Zipper	None	1	3-8	25
3	The Fulcrum	None	1	3-5 each side	33
4	Back Sweep	None	1	5-15	36
5	Crunch and Curl	None	1	10-20	45
6	Twisters	None	1	5-10 each side	62

Special Advanced Techniques

Once you've been training a while, you may want to expand your repertoire. There are many deceptively simple techniques you can use to change the intensity of a single exercise or an entire workout. Learning these techniques increases your options beyond the routines we've laid out for you and helps you further customize your program.

Your middle muscles thrive on change. Presenting them with a variety of stimuli speeds up how fast you see improvements. The beauty of the *Abs of Steel* training system is that it allows you to use the same exercise or exercises and use them in many different ways.

Nearly every exercise in this book includes several variations to help you modify it for your fitness level. There's nothing wrong with sticking with the same basic routines if you like them and you continue to make improvements; however, most people will benefit both mentally and physically by varying their workout. Here are a few more advanced techniques you can use if you wish to spice up your workouts and fine tune your program:

SLOW THINGS DOWN:

Slowing down the speed of each repetition is an excellent way to zero in on your middle muscles. This takes all the momentum out of the movement, so you rely solely on muscle power. The more slowly you perform a rep, the more challenging it is. How slow is slow? Take about five seconds for both the lifting and lowering phase of the move. Because this is an especially potent technique for middle-muscle training, you may need to cut down the number of reps you do per exercise.

PULSES:

Many of the exercises have "pulsing" variations to increase the challenge. A pulse refers to moving up to the top of the movement and then lifting and lowering no more than one or two inches in either direction, 5 to 10 times. Pulses keep continuous tension within the muscles you're working, thereby forcing them to sustain a contraction.

HOLD:

Holding still at the top of a movement has a similar effect as a pulse in that it increases the contraction time of a muscle, and thus builds greater tension within the muscle. This is known as an *isometric hold.* In other instances, holding the exercise in one position for a moment increases the stretch.

SUPER SETS:

When you perform two exercises in a row without any rest in between, this is referred to as a super set. Super sets can be used with two exercises done for the same purpose (for instance, two exercises that isolate your ab muscles) or two exercises that work opposing muscle groups (for example, a lower-back exercise followed by an abdominal exercise or an abdominal exercise followed by a waist exercise). Super sets boost your training intensity by taking away the working muscle's recovery time; it must push extra hard to keep up with the demands placed upon it. For this reason, super setting should only be used by advanced and intermediate exercisers.

GIANT SETS:

Giant sets are exactly what their name implies: three or more exercises strung together in succession with no rest in between. Giant sets work best when they consist only of exercises which isolate that particular muscle group, say your abs or your lower back. Although giant sets are a good way to promote tone and strength, they're only effective if you maintain good form throughout. Only advanced exercisers should utilize this technique.

BLITZ SETS:

Changing the order in which you do your exercises can have a tremendous effect on how your muscles work. It shocks them out of their familiar routine. One way to do a blitz set would be to do your usual routine in the opposite order you normally do it. Another way would be to choose exercises you don't normally do and do them in a completely random order. This system should be used sparingly and only if you've been middle-muscle training for a while. We've outlined the safest, most effective order in which you should do your exercises in the previous chapters. But zapping them with an occasional blitz set may do them some good.

ADDING RESISTANCE:

The problem with adding extra resistance to middle-muscle exercises, in the form of a weight or an exercise band, is that you run the risk of straining your neck and lower back. However, if you are strong enough and are careful to use impeccable form and a slow repetition speed, external weight can definitely be a useful method for increasing the intensity of your target-toning efforts. Begin by a holding the weight against your chest. Once you can easily handle the added weight for the allotted number of reps, try the exercise while gently holding the weight against the top of your head. When that becomes easy, increase the weight. Use very light weights (starting from as little as a half a pound and gradually increasing to three pounds). You may find that holding a weight is too awkward for some exercises.

Exercise bands can also be used to add resistance. Here's an example: wrap a band around a sturdy object such as the leg of a bed or a heavy dresser. Lie down in front of it, hold both ends in one hand, and perform a Reaching Crunch. You will definitely have your abdominal muscles' attention by the tenth rep!

ADDING REPETITIONS:

Once you can do the recommended number of reps per exercise with good form, you can increase the number of reps. Increase gradually, adding no more than two extra reps per exercise per workout. You'll be surprised at what a difference this seemingly small change will make!

Keep in mind, that while a few extra reps will help strengthen and shape your muscles, you can have too much of a good thing. In general, once you can do more than 25 repetitions of a particular exercise, it's time to increase the difficulty level by moving onto a more challenging version, or by trying one of the other special advanced techniques.

Chapter 10

Buns Of Steel

We've included a "bonus" buns chapter because nothing complements ***Abs of Steel*** like a gorgeous pair of buns. A slim, defined middle that tapers into firm, tightly sculpted buns is high on the list of goals for many exercisers. If you are making an effort to strengthen and tone your middle muscles, surely you're willing to invest a little time and energy on your buns, too!

The exercises in this chapter will streamline and define your buns rather than make them bigger and bulkier. Think of these exercises as sort of a lift for the lower body. They will change the contour of your buns by lifting them upward and rounding them into perfect shape. Your buns will look great in everything from a pair of tight jeans to a form-fitting leotard.

The best thing about these exercises and the ***Buns of Steel*** routines at the end of this chapter is how quickly you will see results. No matter what shape you're in when you start, you can create beautifully sculpted buns by following our program. Most women see significant improvements in about a month if they stick with it, faithfully working out two to three times a week. You may feel the benefits even sooner. You know that large hill or flight of stairs you encounter daily? Pretty soon, you'll hop, skip, and bound up to the top with ease!

How To Use These Exercises

At first, you won't need to use weights or any other form of extra resistance to perform most of these exercises. The key is to do each rep with precision so you zero in and target tone your lower-body muscle groups. However, once your muscles grow stronger you will want to move onto the more advanced exercise variations or add additional resistance in the form of a 3- to 8-pound dumbbell or a 1- to 5-pound ankle weight.

Once an exercise becomes too easy, you must change it in order to continue making progress. If you can complete fifteen reps with little effort and while using proper technique, make the exercise more challenging. If, however, you can't complete at least eight repetitions of an exercise without breaking form, it's too difficult. Try a less challenging version of the exercise. If you are already doing an easier version, complete as many reps as you can with good form, rest, and continue when you feel ready.

If you have done very little buns target toning in the past, be sure to rest about ninety seconds between sets. This will give your muscles time to recover so you are not too tired to get the most out of the next set. Gradually cut this rest period down to about thirty seconds—that'll be enough time for you to rest but not so long that you will lose the intensity of the workout.

Consider yourself a beginner and stick with the beginner's buns routines if you haven't done much target toning for your lower body. If you've been target toning between one and three months, start with the intermediate routines; and, if you have been exercising consistently for more than three months, you are probably ready for the advanced routines.

However, these are just guidelines. Your muscles have the ultimate say-so as to whether or not you are working at the proper level! For fastest results, target tone your buns two to three times a week. Do the stretching routine outlined in the *Stretching Out* chapter (p. 64) at the end of every buns workout.

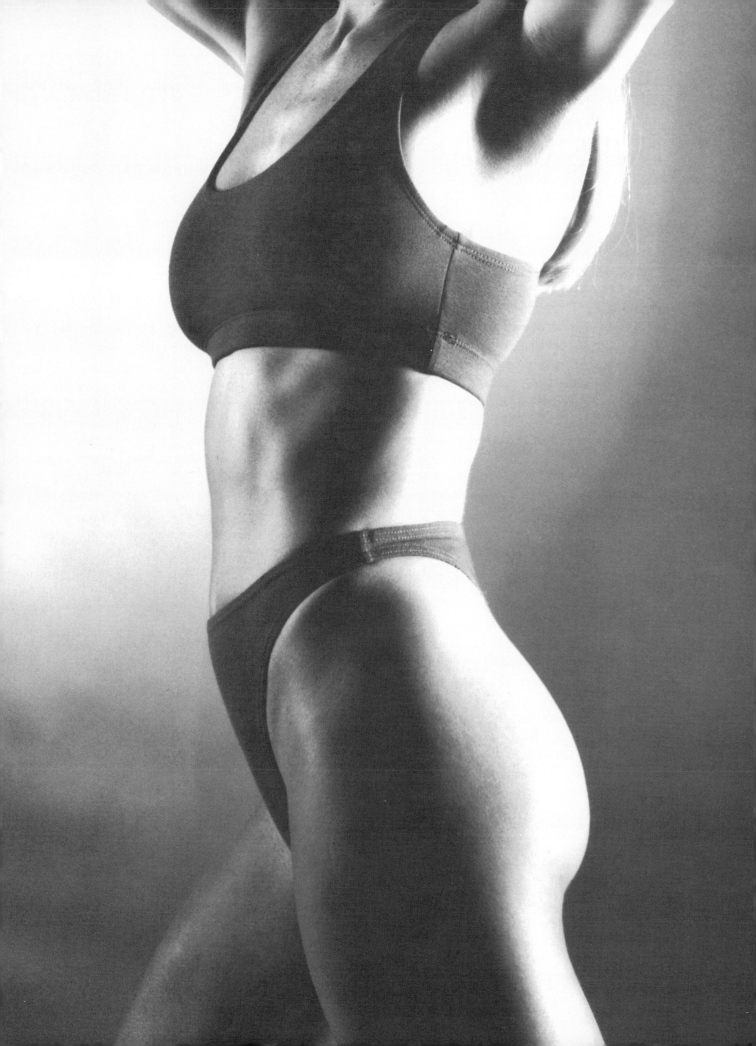

Anatomy

The *gluteus maximus* is your main buns muscle and incidentally, the largest muscle in your body. Its job is to extend your hip. Any time you stand up from a sitting position, climb hills or stairs, or move your leg back behind you, you are using your "glutes." Target toning this muscle will give you a fabulous rear view and complement your newly sculpted abs.

The exercises in this chapter were designed to simultaneously target tone and strengthen the rest of your lower body as you work your glutes—just the way you use your muscles in everyday activities. This promotes a balanced development of your entire lower body so you look firmly proportioned from hip to toe. Here are some of the other major muscle groups you'll work by doing these exercises: your *gluteus medius* and *gluteus minimus*, the muscles located on the outside of your hips; your *quadriceps* and *hamstrings*, your front and back thigh muscles respectively; your *adductors*, the muscles of your inner thighs; and, your *gastrocnemius*, the largest, shapeliest, and most powerful of your calf muscles.

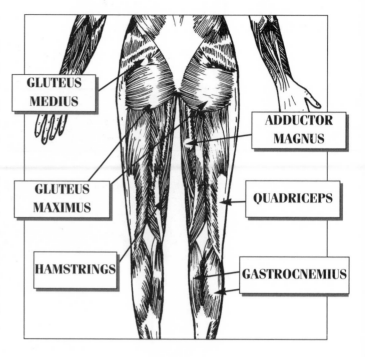

The Exercises In This Chapter

1. Static Bun Lifts
2. Squats
3. Dips
4. Back Lunges with Bun Sweeps
5. Single Leg Squats
6. Bun Presses with Band
7. Wall Sit-Pelvic Tilt Combo
8. Turned Out Leg Lifts

Static Bun Lifts

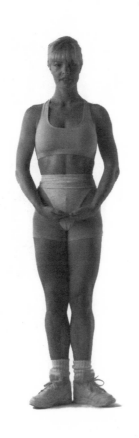

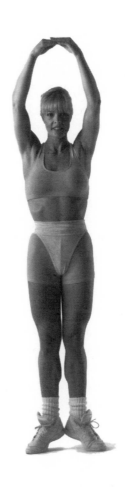

SET-UP:

Stand tall with your heels together and your toes angled slightly outward. Firmly squeeze your buns and thighs together. Lightly clasp your hands together and rest them on top of your thighs. Pull your abs inward and maintain natural alignment.

MOVE:

Squeeze your buns and thighs together even more firmly as you raise your heels off the floor and lift your arms up over your head. Hold a moment and return to the start.

MIND BODY CONNECTION:

Use the lifting of your arms to remind yourself to pull up straight and tall. You'll feel this in your buns, inner and outer thighs, and lower legs, especially as you raise your heels up off the floor. This exercise is useful to teach you how to contract your buns muscles when you're doing other buns exercises.

VARIATIONS:

- To increase the intensity of this move, pulse 5 to10 times in the up position by raising and lowering your heels a small distance.
- Add extra resistance by holding a one- to three-pound dumbbell in each hand.
- To decrease the intensity of this move, separate your heels about half an inch.

FORM TIPS:

- Don't allow your heels to lose contact with each other, especially as you lower to the start.
- Maintain a tall and aligned posture.
- Keep your neck and shoulders relaxed, especially as you lift your arms.

Squats

SET-UP:

Stand tall with your feet hip-width apart, with your hands on your hips. Broaden your chest by relaxing your shoulders backward and downward and keeping your rib cage lifted. Pull your abdominals gently inward and maintain a natural curve in your spine.

MOVE:

Leading with your tailbone, sit backward and downward until your thighs are parallel to the floor; slide your hands onto your thighs as you lower. As you hold for a moment in the lowered position, squeeze your buns together. Return to the starting position by pressing up through your heels.

MIND BODY CONNECTION:

Pretend your tailbone is sliding along an imaginary wall directly behind you. You should feel the muscles in your buns and in front of your thighs contract, especially as you squeeze and return to the starting position.

VARIATIONS:

- To place greater emphasis on your inner thighs, do a plié, standing with your legs slightly wider than hip-width apart and your toes angled outward. Squat until your thighs are parallel to the floor.
- Add extra resistance by holding a dumbbell in each hand with your arms down at your sides or placing a light barbell across your shoulders.
- If you find this move too difficult, or if it causes discomfort in your knees, only squat a quarter to one half way to parallel.

FORM TIPS:

- Your knees should never travel forward of your toes so don't allow your thighs to go lower than parallel.
- Be careful not to overarch your lower back or lean too far forward.
- As you move upward, don't "lock" your knees by straightening them all the way; they should be slightly bent at the top of the movement.

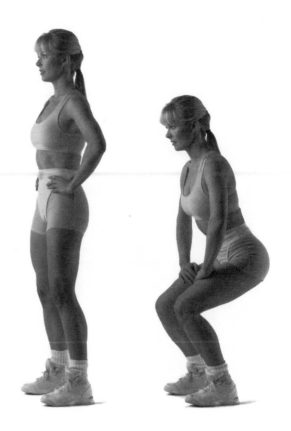

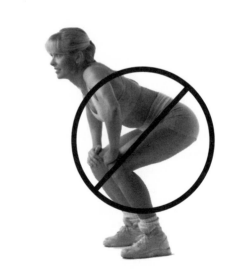

FOCUS ON FORM:

Don't squat below parallel or lean too far forward! Your knees should never move out past your toes and you should always maintain good upper-body alignment.

Dips

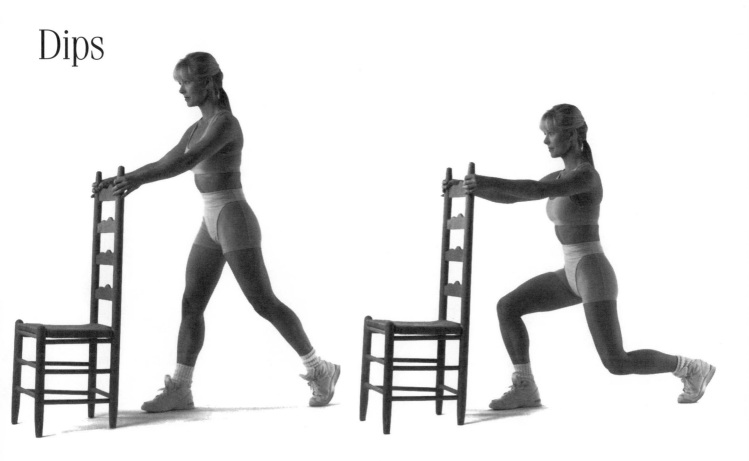

SET-UP:

Stand with your feet hip-width apart and step your left foot back about a stride's length until your legs are about three feet apart in a "straddled" position. Bend your front knee slightly and lift your back heel off the floor. Pull your abs inward and lift up tall. With both hands, hold onto a stable object in front or hold on with one hand that is placed to the side.

MOVE:

Bend both knees so that your back knee almost, but not quite, touches the floor. In the lowered position, your back knee will point directly down toward the floor, and your front thigh will be parallel to it. Hold a moment and return to the start. Switch legs and do an equal number of reps.

MIND BODY CONNECTION:

Imagine you are on a balance beam and must dip straight down with perfect alignment in order not to fall off. You'll feel this move in your buns and thighs, especially as you push upward.

VARIATIONS:

If this exercise isn't challenging enough:

- Try placing your hands on your hips.
- Hold a dumbbell in each hand with your arms down at your sides.
- Do a Basic Lunge: start with your feet hip-width apart. Leading with your heel, step forward about a stride length into the starting Dip position. Dip down, straighten your legs, and then step back to the start. Do an equal number of reps with both legs.

FORM TIPS:

- Don't allow your front knee to travel in front of your toes as you lower.
- Be careful not to fully straighten your knees or bend so far forward from the waist that you feel off balance.
- Maintain good upper-body alignment.

Back Lunges with Bun Sweeps

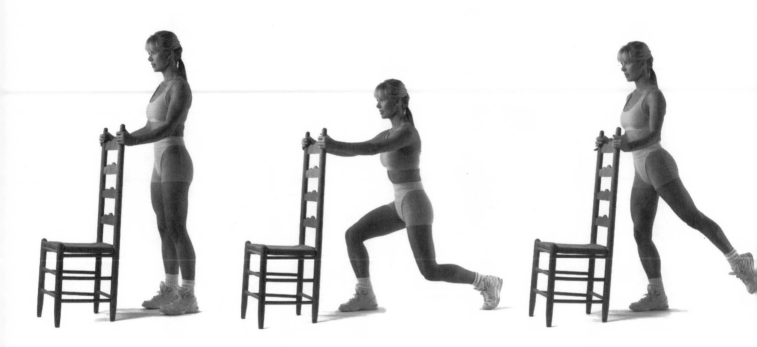

SET-UP:
Stand tall with your feet hip-width apart. Pull your abdominals gently in toward your spine and maintain a natural alignment. Hold onto a sturdy object with both hands for support.

MOVE:
Step your left foot backward about a stride's length and bend both knees until your left thigh is pointing straight down toward the floor and your right thigh is parallel to it. Land softly on the ball of your left foot, keeping your heel up. Then, push upward and, as you straighten your left leg, sweep it backward and upward a few inches until you feel a contraction through your buns. Hold a moment and step back to the start. Switch legs and do an equal number of reps.

MIND BODY CONNECTION:
Pretend you are stepping on an object directly behind you and then sweeping it up and away with your foot. You will feel this move in your buns, thighs, and lower leg, especially as you stand up and sweep your leg backward.

VARIATIONS:
- If you find this exercise too hard to do, omit the Bun Sweep or do it as a separate exercise.
- If you want to make this exercise a bit more difficult, don't hold onto the chair for support.
- For a real challenge, hold the top position of the Bun Sweep and pulse your leg 5 to 10 times by squeezing your buns and pressing your foot a short way forward and back.

FORM TIPS:
- Don't overstep the Back Lunge phase so much that you lose your balance and alignment.
- When your foot contacts the floor, it should land softly and noiselessly.
- Don't sweep your foot so far back and up that you arch your back.

Single Leg Squats

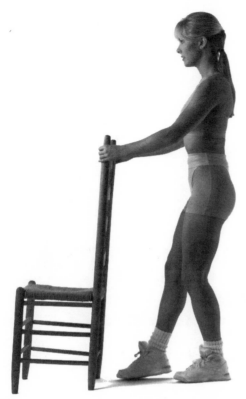

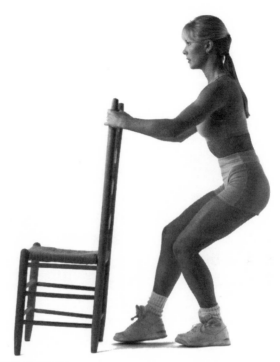

SET-UP:

Stand tall, about an arm's length away from a sturdy chair; hold onto it with your hands for support. Extend your right leg a small way in front of you with a slightly bent knee; lift your right heel and inside edge of your foot a short distance off the floor. Sit back into your left leg so that most of your weight is supported on it.

MOVE:

While maintaining good posture, bend your left knee about six inches and lower your body a few inches toward the floor; your right leg will remain stationary. As you hold a moment, squeeze your buns together. Return to the start, taking care not to fully lock your knees. Switch legs and do an equal number of repetitions.

MIND BODY CONNECTION:

To get the most from this exercise do it slowly: move down for a slow two count and then up for a slow two count. You're doing it right when you feel the muscles in the front of your thigh contracting both on the way up and the way down.

VARIATIONS:

- If you find this exercise too easy, lift your right foot up a few inches off the floor as you lower into the Squat position.
- To add resistance, hold a dumbbell in the hand on the opposite side of your working leg.
- If you find this exercise too difficult, only bend your knee about three inches.

FORM TIPS:

- Stand up tall and keep your abs pulled in throughout.
- You will not be able to squat as low as you can when you do a Basic Squat.

Bun Presses with Band

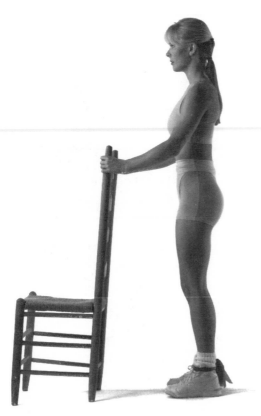
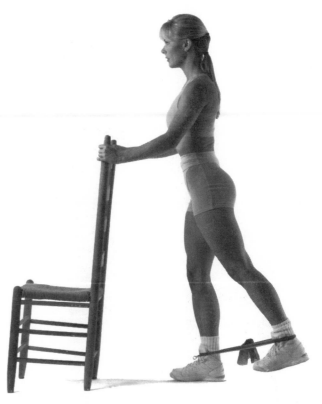

SET-UP:

Securely tie together the two ends of about two feet of an exercise band or tube to make a closed loop and place it around both of your ankles. Stand tall with your feet hip-width apart, toes facing forward. Hold onto a stable object such as sturdy chair for support. Tighten your abdominals, and maintain a natural body alignment.

THE MOVE:

Squeeze your buns together and kick your left foot directly back behind you until the band is taut, and you feel a contraction in your buns. Hold a moment and return to the start. Switch working legs and then do an equal number of reps with your right foot.

MIND BODY CONNECTION:

This is a very small, precise movement. If you keep constant tension on the band, you will feel continuous tension in your buns and down the back of your thigh.

VARIATIONS:

- To make this move more advanced, pulse 5 to 10 times a few inches up and down at the top of the movement or use an exercise band which provides more resistance.
- If this move is too difficult, do it without the band around your ankles.

FORM TIPS:

- To avoid overarching your lower back, don't press your leg too far back.
- Good posture is the key to making this exercise most effective. If you slouch or lean forward from the waist, your buns won't receive an effective workout.

Wall Sit-Pelvic Tilt Combo

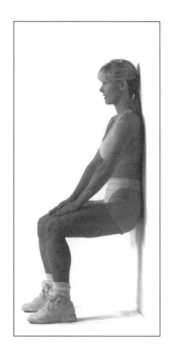

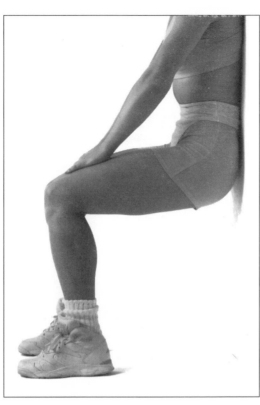

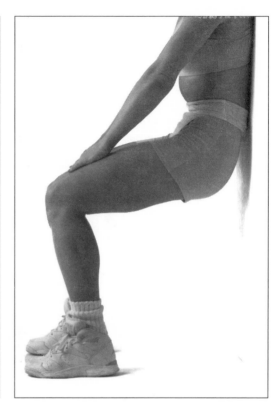

SET-UP:

Stand with your back against a wall with your arms at your sides and place your feet hip-width apart and about a foot away from the wall. Maintain good posture by keeping your spine naturally aligned, your shoulders relaxed, and your abdominals pulled inward. Slide your body down along the wall until your hips are in line with your knees, and your thighs are parallel to the floor.

MOVE:

While holding the Wall Sit position, gently squeeze your buns together and tilt your pelvis forward so that your buns curl off the wall slightly and your hip bones travel forward. Hold a moment and repeat. Complete all reps before sliding up and back into the starting position.

MIND BODY CONNECTION:

Pretend you're sitting in a chair and trying to slide yourself forward to the edge of the seat. You will immediately feel tension in the tops of your thighs as you move into the seated position; this tension will grow stronger as you hold the Wall Sit. You will feel a strong contraction in your buns both from holding the Wall Sit and from performing the Pelvic Tilt.

VARIATIONS:

If you find this exercise too difficult:

• Omit the Pelvic Tilt or do it while lying on your back as a separate exercise.

• Only lower yourself a quarter to one half of the fully seated position.

FORM TIPS:

• Your alignment is correct if there is a very slight gap between the small of your back and the wall. Avoid sitting too low; don't allow your hips to move below parallel or your knees to travel forward of your toes.

• If you have a history of high blood pressure, limit your time in the Wall Sit position to no more than ten seconds at a time (about three Pelvic Tilts). You can complete repetitions by doing several sets.

• Do not hold your breath!

Turned Out Leg Lifts

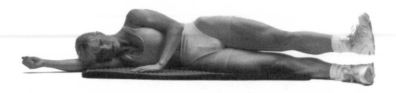

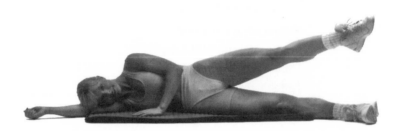

SET-UP:
Lie on your right side with your back and buns along the back edge of your exercise mat with your legs straight and about six inches forward of your hips. Align your top hip directly over your bottom hip and turn your left knee up to the ceiling by squeezing your buns together and rotating your left hip outward. Place your left palm on the floor in front of your chest for support and rest your head on your outstretched right arm.

MOVE:
Flex your left foot and, leading with your toe, lift your leg a few inches higher than shoulder height. Point your toe and then lower your leg, with resistance, to the start. Flex your foot once again before beginning the next rep. Switch sides and do an equal number of reps with the right leg.

MIND BODY CONNECTION:
As you lower your leg, pretend you are trying to resist the weight of a heavy sandbag. Pointing your toe as you lower will help you concentrate on lengthening your leg, turning your knee upward, and squeezing your buns. You will feel this in your outer hip, buns, and thighs. Pointing and flexing your foot works your calf muscles.

VARIATIONS:
*   Once you have completed half the number of repetitions for that set, complete the remaining reps by pointing your toe as you lift and flexing your foot as you lower. This will increase the intensity of the exercise.
*   For resistance, add an ankle weight.
*   To make this exercise less challenging, bend your working leg slightly.

FORM TIPS:
*   Pull your abs inward and align your neck with the rest of your spine. This will prevent your top hip from rolling backward.

Buns Routines

Here are three buns routines you can try. Figure out how much time you want to spend target toning your buns (5, 15, or 20 minutes) and then adapt that routine to your level. Once you've tried our routines for a while, feel free to make up your own.

5-Minute Routines

BEGINNER

Order	Exercise	Resistance/Variation	Sets	Reps	Page
1	Static Bun Lifts	None	1	8-15	97
2	Squats	None	1	8-15	98
3	Dips	None	1	8-15	99
4	Turned Out Leg Lifts	None	1	8-15	104

INTERMEDIATE

Order	Exercise	Resistance/Variation	Sets	Reps	Page
1	Static Bun Lifts	Pulse 5-10 times at top	1	8-15	97
2	Squats	Dumbbells	1	8-15	98
3	Dips	Dumbbells	1	8-15	99
4	Turned Out Leg Lifts	None	1	8-15	104

ADVANCED

Order	Exercise	Resistance/Variation	Sets	Reps	Page
1	Static Bun Lifts	Dumbbells; pulse 5-10 times at top	1	8-15	97
2	Squats	Dumbbells; do plié version for one set	1	8-15	98
3	Dips	Do Basic Lunge version	1	8-15	99
4	Turned Out Leg Lifts	Ankle weight	1	8-15	104

15-Minute Routines

BEGINNER

Order	Exercise	Resistance/Variation	Sets	Reps	Page
1	Static Bun Lifts	None	1	8-15	97
2	Squats	None	2	8-15	98
3	Dips	None	1	8-15	99
4	Back Lunges w/Bun Sweeps	None	1	8-15	100
5	Bun Presses w/Band	None	1	8-15	102
6	Turned Out Leg Lifts	None	1	8-15	104

INTERMEDIATE

Order	Exercise	Resistance/Variation	Sets	Reps	Page
1	Static Bun Lifts	Dumbbells	1	8-15	97
2	Squats	Dumbbells	2	8-15	98
3	Dips	None	1	8-15	99
4	Single Leg Squats	None	1	8-15	101
5	Back Lunges w/Bun Sweeps	None	1	8-15	100
6	Bun Presses w/Band	Exercise band	1	8-15	102
7	Turned Out Leg Lifts	Ankle Weight	1	8-15	104

ADVANCED

Order	Exercise	Resistance/Variation	Sets	Reps	Page
1	Static Bun Lifts	Dumbbells; pulse 5-10 times at top	1	8-15	97
2	Squats	Dumbbells	2	8-15	98
3	Dips	Dumbbells; do Basic Lunge version	1	8-15	99
4	Single Leg Squats	Lift opposite foot up	1	8-15	101
5	Back Lunges w/Bun Sweeps	Pulse 5-10 times at top	1	8-15	100
6	Bun Presses w/Band	With band, pulse 5-10 times at top	1	8-15	102
7	Wall Sit-Pelvic Tilt Combo	None	1	8-15	103
8	Turned Out Leg Lifts	Ankle weight; alternate point/flex	1	8-15	104

20-Minute Routines

BEGINNER

Order	Exercise	Resistance/Variation	Sets	Reps	Page
1	Static Bun Lifts	None	2	8-15	97
2	Squats	None	2	8-15	98
3	Dips	None	2	8-15	99
4	Single Leg Squats	None	1	8-15	101
5	Back Lunges w/Bun Sweeps	None	1	8-15	100
6	Bun Presses w/Band	None	2	8-15	102
7	Wall Sit-Pelvic Tilt Combo	None	1	8-15	103
8	Turned Out Leg Lifts	None	2	8-15	104

INTERMEDIATE

Order	Exercise	Resistance/Variation	Sets	Reps	Page
1	Static Bun Lifts	Dumbbells	2	8-15	97
2	Squats	Dumbbells for one set, plié version one set	2	8-15	98
3	Dips	Do second set as Basic Lunge	2	8-15	99
4	Single Leg Squats	None	1	8-15	101
5	Back Lunges w/Bun Sweeps	None	1	8-15	100
6	Bun Presses w/Band	With exercise band, pulse 5-10 times at top for one set	2	8-15	102
7	Wall Sit-Pelvic Tilt Combo	None	1	8-15	103
8	Turned Out Leg Lifts	Alternate point/flex for one set	2	8-15	104

ADVANCED

Order	Exercise	Resistance/Variation	Sets	Reps	Page
1	Static Bun Lifts	Dumbbells; pulse 5-10 times at top for one set	2	8-15	97
2	Squats	Dumbbells for one set, plié version one set	2	8-15	98
3	Dips	Dumbbells; do second set as Basic Lunge	2	8-15	99
4	Single Leg Squats	Lift opposite foot up	1	8-15	101
5	Back Lunges w/Bun Sweeps	Pulse 5-10 times at top	1	8-15	100
6	Bun Presses w/Band	With exercise band, pulse 5-10 times at top for one set	2	8-15	102
7	Wall Sit-Pelvic Tilt Combo	None	2	8-15	103
8	Turned Out Leg Lifts	Ankle weight; alternate point/flex	1	8-15	104

Glossary

Abdominals: Usually refers to the *rectus abdominis* muscle, a flat, wide sheet of muscle which attaches to your rib cage, runs the length of your torso, and attaches to your pelvis. This muscle flexes (curls) and stabilizes the spine. It's best worked with crunches and stabilization and awareness exercises.

Advanced Exerciser: Someone who scores an advanced rating on the middle-muscle strength and flexibility tests and who can perform the majority of the advanced variations of the middle-muscles, target-toning exercises. Usually, this is someone who has been regularly participating in a middle-muscle, target-toning program for three months or more.

Aerobic Exercise: Sustained exercise such as walking, running, or cycling, which requires oxygen for fuel. Involves the repetitive, rhythmic movement of large muscle groups such as your buns and thighs and causes an elevation in heart rate. The most efficient calorie and fat burning form of exercise.

Alignment: Refers to posture. Natural alignment is an ideal posture in which your head is centered between your shoulders, your shoulders are relaxed backward and downward, your chest and rib cage are lifted, your abdominals are pulled in towards your spine, your lower body is relaxed, and your weight is distributed evenly on both feet.

Anaerobic Exercise: Short bursts of exercise, usually lasting less than a minute, designed to increase the power, strength, and tone of a muscle. It relies on cellular enzymes rather than oxygen for fuel. Example: target toning.

Beginning Exerciser: Someone who scores a beginner's rating on the middle-muscle strength and flexibility tests, and who finds the basic versions of most middle-muscle, target-toning exercises a challenge. Usually, this is someone who has not been regularly participating in a middle-muscle, target-toning program or who has participated in a low intensity routine.

Blitz Set: An advanced technique which calls for mixing up the order of exercises and changing the exercises you normally do. This stimulates your middle muscles to tighten and tone.

Body Fat Percentage: A method of determining body composition: how much of your weight is fat and how much is lean body tissue, or muscle. Optimal body fat percentages for women are between 16 and 26 percent; for men, 12 to 20 percent.

Body Weight: Your weight in pounds. Usually taken on a scale. This is not a good determinant of fitness because it does not distinguish how much of your body composition is fat and how much is muscle.

Buns: Your *gluteus maximus* muscle, which gives your rear end its rounded shape. The *gluteus medius* and *minimus* shape the sides of your buns. Best worked with exercises in the bonus *Buns of Steel* chapter.

Carbohydrate: Your body's main nutritional energy source. Simple carbohydrates include sugars, candies, cakes, and cookies. They're low in nutritional value and provide quick energy. Complex carbs include grains, cereals, and vegetables. They are good sources of nutrition and long-term energy. Between 55 and 65 percent of your daily intake should come from carbohydrates.

Cardiovascular Exercise: Aerobic exercise which works the heart and lungs, and, if done on a regular basis, increases endurance and the efficiency of oxygen use.

Contraction: When a muscle responds to a force by shortening, lengthening, or pushing against it without changing length. A contraction is experienced in the form of tension in the muscle being worked.

Cool Down: A period immediately following heavy exercise during which light activity such as slow walking and stretching is done in order to allow your heart rate, blood pressure, and body temperature to lower.

Definition: Having a degree of muscular development which shows through the skin due to a low amount of body fat. Also known as muscularity, cut up, sculpted, or chiseled.

Dumbbell: A short-handled weight bar used to add resistance to an exercise. A "free weight."

Exercise: Refers to the actual movement you are doing in a workout. For instance, a Basic Crunch in an abdominals workout or a Squat in a buns workout.

Exercise Band or Tube: A sturdy elastic band or tube designed specifically to add resistance to an exercise. With or without handles. Some brand names include Dynabands, Exer-tubing, and Spri. (Surgical tubing may be used as a suitable substitute.)

Extension: An increase in the angle of a joint. In the case of your spine, this refers to any backward bending or arching movement.

Fat: A nutritional energy source for your body. Sources include oils, marbled meat, nuts, seeds, butter, eggs. No more than 20 to 25 percent of your daily intake should come from dietary fat. (Also see *Body Fat Percentage.*)

Fitness: The body's ability to function optimally. Fitness level refers to your present level of physical condition.

Flexibility: Refers to the degree of mobility or the range of motion through which a joint can move. A consistent program of stretching exercises increases flexibility.

Flexion: A decrease in the angle of a joint. In the case of your spine, this refers to any forward bending, curling, or crunching movement.

Giant Set: A technique that involves combining three or more sets of different exercises with no rest in between.

Holds: A method of increasing intensity by holding an exercise at the top of a movement. This is an isometric technique (the muscle does not change its length) which increases the duration that a muscle contracts. In other instances, holding increases the amount of stretch you experience.

Intensity: The quality of effort you put into a workout or individual exercise.

Intermediate Exerciser: Someone who has scored an intermediate rating on the middle-muscle strength and flexibility tests and who can easily complete the basic versions of most target-toning exercises but can not yet complete the more advanced versions without undue strain or diminished technique. Usually, this is someone who has been regularly participating in a target-toning program for between one and three months.

Lower Back: Refers to the *erector spinae* muscles which attach to the back of your spine and are responsible for extending (backward bending) and stabilizing your spine. These muscles are best worked with stabilization and awareness exercises and lower-back stretching and strengthening exercises.

Middle Muscles: Refers to a combination of all the muscles that wrap around your torso and which are responsible for supporting and moving your spine. These include: your abs (*transversus* and *rectus abdominis*), waist (*internal* and *external obliques*), and lower-back (*erector spinae*) muscles.

Mind Body Connection: Something that helps link your thought process with your body's movement. Often this is done by relating the movement to something that is familiar.

Program: An entire exercise schedule, as in the **Abs of Steel** middle-muscle workout program.

Protein: A nutritional element your body uses to build and repair muscle and to a limited extent, as an energy source. Dietary sources include lean meats and poultry, fish, legumes, and vegetables. About 15 to 20 percent of your daily intake should come from protein.

Pulse: A method of increasing the intensity of an

exercise by moving to the top of the movement and then lifting and lowering it a very small distance, usually no more than one or two inches in either direction. This puts continuous tension on the muscle by forcing it to sustain a contraction.

Repetition: A complete movement of an exercise. Also: rep. Plural: reps.

Resistance: Something that places a force, or tension, on a muscle. This can be external, such as a weight or exercise band, or something as simple as gravity of your own body weight.

Rest: The briefest possible interval between sets, which allows the working muscle to regain strength. Also: the time interval between workouts.

Routine: A group of exercises.

Set: A group of continuously performed repetitions of an exercise.

Soft: Not fully straightened or "locked," as it applies to a joint such as the knee or elbow.

Split Routine: A method of training in which different muscle groups are target toned on different days.

Spot Reducing: A misnomer. You cannot selectively lose fat on any part of your body. However, you can target tone a specific muscle or muscle group (see *Target Toning*).

Stabilization and Awareness: Any exercise which utilizes your middle muscles to support and protect your spine or which makes you more aware of the proper movement of your spine. Stabilization and awareness exercises work your middle muscles three-dimensionally; that is, they use all your middle muscles simultaneously, as a team.

Super Set: A technique that involves combining two sets of two different exercises with no rest in between.

Target Toning: A method of training that utilizes resistance and precise, focused movements to bring about increases in tone, definition, and muscular strength.

Training Variable: A workout element which can be adjusted in order to increase or decrease the intensity of your program.

Vertebrae: The individual bones which, together, form your spinal column. There are 24 vertebrae.

Waist: A term which refers to the most tapered part of your torso; where your *internal* and *external oblique* muscles wrap around your middle. These muscles are responsible for flexing (curling) and stabilizing the spine as well as any twisting or side bending movements of the spine. They're best worked with exercises like those in the *Your Waist* chapter.

Warm-Up: The period of time where you engage in light activities such as walking or easy jogging in order to prepare your body for hard physical exercise. The warm-up period increases the blood flow to your muscles, speeds up heart rate, and elevates body temperature.

INDEX

Biographies

LEISA HART, a fitness professional for the past ten years, is the star of more than a dozen *Buns of Steel* videos. She is an *American Council of Exercise* certified personal trainer and co-author of *Buns of Steel: Total Body Workout* and the *Buns of Steel Cookbook*. She represents several innovative fitness products, including the *Buns Worker* by *Fitness Quest*, *MET-Rx*, and *National Laboratories* vitamins, and is the owner of *The Fitness Edge Health Club* in Dallas, Texas.

LIZ NEPORENT has a master's degree in exercise physiology and is certified by the *American College of Sports Medicine*, the *American Council on Exercise*, and the *National Strength and Conditioning Association*. She is president of *Frontline Fitness*, a New York-based corporate consulting company and is co-author of *Buns of Steel: Total Body Workout* and *The Crunch Fitness Workout*.

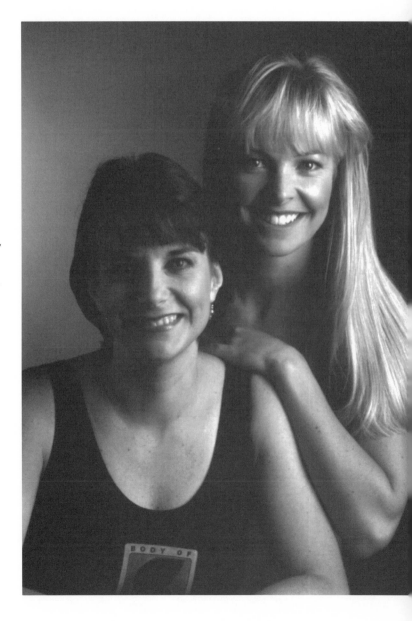

HERE ARE SOME MORE SECRET INGREDIENTS FOR GREAT ABS!

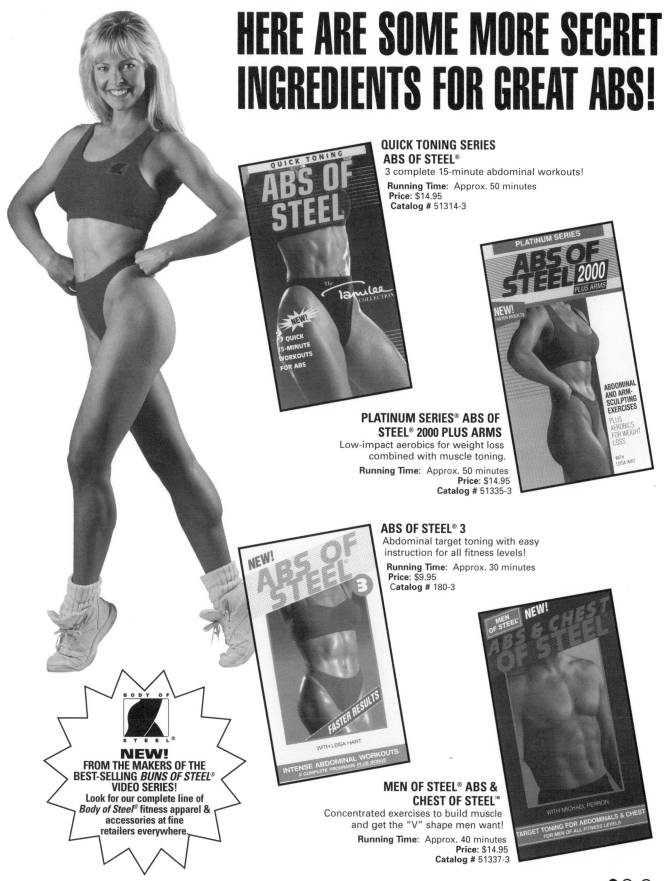

QUICK TONING SERIES
ABS OF STEEL®
3 complete 15-minute abdominal workouts!

Running Time: Approx. 50 minutes
Price: $14.95
Catalog # 51314-3

PLATINUM SERIES® ABS OF STEEL® 2000 PLUS ARMS
Low-impact aerobics for weight loss combined with muscle toning.

Running Time: Approx. 50 minutes
Price: $14.95
Catalog # 51335-3

ABS OF STEEL® 3
Abdominal target toning with easy instruction for all fitness levels!

Running Time: Approx. 30 minutes
Price: $9.95
Catalog # 180-3

MEN OF STEEL® ABS & CHEST OF STEEL™
Concentrated exercises to build muscle and get the "V" shape men want!

Running Time: Approx. 40 minutes
Price: $14.95
Catalog # 51337-3

NEW!
FROM THE MAKERS OF THE BEST-SELLING *BUNS OF STEEL®* VIDEO SERIES!
Look for our complete line of *Body of Steel®* fitness apparel & accessories at fine retailers everywhere.

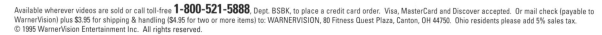